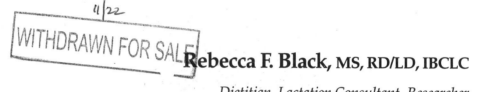

LACTATION SPECIALIST SELF-STUDY SERIES

Module 2
The Process of Breastfeeding

Rebecca F. Black, MS, RD/LD, IBCLC

Dietitian, Lactation Consultant, Researcher
President, Augusta Nutrition Consultants
Augusta, Georgia

Leasa Jarman, MS

Education Consultant
Augusta, Georgia

Jan B. Simpson, RN, BSN, IBCLC

Nurse, Lactation Consultant
Tuscaloosa, Alabama

JONES AND BARTLETT PUBLISHERS
Sudbury, Massachusetts

BOSTON   TORONTO   LONDON   SINGAPORE

World Headquarters
Jones and Bartlett Publishers
40 Tall Pine Drive
Sudbury, MA 01776
978 443-5000
info@jbpub.com
www.jbpub.com

Jones and Bartlett Publishers Canada
2100 Bloor St. West
Suite #6-272
Toronto, ON M6S 5A5

Jones and Bartlett Publishers International
Barb House, Barb Mews
London W6 7PA
UK

Cover illustration is a woodcut print by Russell Wray, Gull Rock Pottery, 325 East Side Road, Hancock, ME 04640.

Acknowledgment: Supported in part through funds from the Georgia WIC Program, Maternal and Child Health Branch, Division of Public Health, Georgia Department of Human Resources.

Library of Congress Cataloging-in-Publication Data
The process of breastfeeding / edited by Rebecca F. Black, Leasa Jarman, Jan B. Simpson.
      p.   cm.—(Lactation specialist self-study series : module 2)
      Includes bibliographical references.
      ISBN 0-7637-0195-5 (alk. paper)
      1. Breast feeding—Study and teaching.   I. Black, Rebecca F.
II. Jarman, Leasa.   III. Simpson, Jan B.   IV. Series.
RJ216.S885   1997
613.2'69--dc21   97-25569
                                                CIP

Editor: Robin Carter
Production Editor: Joan M. Flaherty
Editorial Production Service: Marilyn E. Rash
Design/Typesetting: Ruth Maassen
Cover Design: Hannus Design Associates
Cover Illustration: Russell Wray
Cover Printing: Malloy Lithographing
Printing and Binding: Malloy Lithographing

Printed in the United States of America
01 00 99   10 9 8 7 6 5 4 3 2

Contents

Preface

Lactation consultants number in the thousands; they represent the varied disciplines of counseling, education, nursing, nutrition, occupational therapy, pharmacy, physical therapy, psychology, and medicine. The differing backgrounds of lactation consultants and the lack of a widespread educational program of study for lactation consulting results in professionals with strengths in particular areas of lactation. As we enter the next millenium, and possibly more control of healthcare resources by managed care and less choice by the consumer, it is imperative that those in lactation consulting share a base knowledge from many disciplines to compete and survive. As resources shrink, health-care professionals must expand their clinical skills to improve their marketability. Because boundaries separating prenatal, hospital, and postpartum services are becoming less defined, organizations and hospitals strive to compete for services outside their traditional roles.

The Lactation Specialist Self-Study Series draws extensively from the literature of all related disciplines. It is designed in four separate modules to present a systematic overview of the profession (support, process, science, and management of breastfeeding), emphasizing and reviewing areas for study usually lacking in the academic preparation of nurses and nutritionists. *The Process of Breastfeeding*, Module 2 of *The Lactation Specialist Self-Study Series*, explores the initiation and assessment of lactation, common problems in breastfeeding, breastmilk expression, and accessory items available to promote successful breastfeeding.

Chapter 1 on initiating and assessing lactation has three sections: preparing to breastfeed, feeding at the breast, and breastfeeding assessment. Emphasis is placed on ways to provide prenatal breastfeeding education, early breast assessment and treatment to identify breast or nipple and areolar abnormalities that may hinder breastfeeding, and nipple and breast care. The section on feeding at the breast discusses the mother's and infant's readiness to feed, early feedings, cueing, positioning, and latching techniques. The third section of the chapter reviews breastfeeding assessment, including the individual feed and the process of breastfeeding over time. Tools to document and evaluate feeding are presented from the literature.

The second chapter on common problems includes four sections: structural elements of the areolar and nipple tissue with an emphasis on wound healing, nipple soreness, breast-related problems, and infant-related problems. Only the more common situations seen in daily practice are reviewed in this chapter, reserving the more unusual situations for discussion in Module 4 of this series, *The Management of Breastfeeding*.

The final chapter of this module covers the manual and mechanical expression of breastmilk, human milk banks, and breastfeeding accessories, such as nursing supplementer devices, bra pads, breast shells and shields, creams and ointments, and nursing pillows and fashions. A resource listing by item is provided at the end of this chapter.

The format of the module is designed to be reader-friendly, with pre- and post-test questions for each section, extensive reference lists, and a useful index. There are 360 multiple-choice questions in *The Process of Breastfeeding*—the pre- and post-test format helps the learner gauge his or her knowledge about the content covered prior to and after completion of a section. The format easily lends itself to use in a formal learning environment, such as an undergraduate or graduate curriculum, or for the student or clinician looking for a systematic way to prepare for the profession or obtain informal continuing education.

Acknowledgments

In 1992, the state of Georgia public health nutrition section identified the need to update the knowledge and skills of practicing nurses and nutritionists in the field of lactation. The *Lactation Specialist Self-Study Series* was first developed as an eleven-volume set of modules and was supported in part through funds from the Georgia WIC Program, Maternal and Child Health Branch, Division of Public Health, Georgia Department of Human Resources. Many individuals were instrumental in the early development of the series. I wish to thank Carol McGowan for her vision of the project and the faith that the project would finally come to fruition, Gwen Gustavson for her pilot teaching of the curricula to nutritionists in two health districts in Georgia, and Irene Frei and Frances Wilkinson for their support of the project by providing the needed resources.

Many other individuals have helped this *Series* become a reality: Tracy Howie and Jerry Smith were invaluable for their technical computer expertise; Debi Bocar, Martha Brower, and Julie Stock reviewed all four modules and provided excellent suggestions about them for continuing education applications as well as feedback for improvement; Jatinder Bhatia and Elizabeth Williams also provided valuable constructive feedback from the medical community about selected modules.

I would be remiss if I failed to thank the behind-the-scene supportive individuals who kept my business running for what, at times, must have seemed like forever. Emily Kitchens, my business manager, is invaluable to me and without her organizational abilities, tireless energy, and loyalty Augusta Nutrition Consultants, Inc., would fold. The lactation consultants and peer counselors on staff filled in for me in many situations and provided valuable insight for the *Series*. Many dietetic interns enrolled in the Augusta Area Dietetic Internship combed the library in search of articles as did Donna Wilson. The librarians at the Medical College of Georgia never wearied of my requests for reprints and seemingly daily presence on the Medline. Thanks also goes to the nutrition and pediatric professors at the Medical College of Georgia School of Medicine and Graduate School for their willingness to answer questions and interpret literature.

Jan Simpson, one of the editors, was very instrumental in the *Lactation Specialist Self-Study Series*. Not only did she write several of the chapters but she also helped in the development of the content of the modules as well as the completion of the applications for nursing continuing education credits. Jan and her family worked many hours to get the *Series* finished. Leasa Jarman, another editor, provided expertise on test construction and evaluated each module for completeness of the objectives and each test for accurate measurement of the objectives. Thanks also to the individual contributors who are too numerous to mention here but are all named on the Contributors' list.

I wish to thank my family—Tony, Helen, and Marie—who gave so willingly of Mom and accompanied me on several trips to educational workshops. Many evening hours and weekends were lost to the *Series* and their support was essential to its successful completion. Finally, I wish to acknowledge the presence and guidance of the Lord Jesus Christ who gives me the strength to press on to the prize of eternal life through Him.

Rebecca Black

Lactation Specialist Self-Study Series

Contributors

Rebecca F. Black, MS, RD/LD, IBCLC
President, Augusta Nutrition
   Consultants, Inc.
Augusta, Georgia

Donna Calhoun, BS, IBCLC
Lactation Consultant
Breast Expressions
Augusta, Georgia

Leasa Jarman, MS
Educator
Columbia County School System
Augusta, Georgia

Jan B. Simpson, RN, BSN, IBCLC
Lactation Consultant in Private
   Practice
Tuscaloosa, Alabama

Martha K. Grodrian, RD, LD, IBCLC
Dayton, Ohio

Pamela D. Hill, PhD, RN
Chicago, Illinois

Kathleen E. Huggins, RN, MS
San Luis Obispo, California

Karen Sanders Moore, RNC, MSN, IBCLC
Saint Louis, Missouri

Julie Stock, MA, IBCLC
Chicago, Illinois

Elizabeth Williams, MD, MPH, IBCLC
Stanford, California

Reviewers

Debi Leslie Bocar, RN, MEd, MS, IBCLC
Oklahoma City, Oklahoma

CHAPTER 1

Initiating and Assessing Lactation

SECTION A

Preparing to Breastfeed

Rebecca F. Black, MS, RD/LD, IBCLC
Donna Calhoun, BS, IBCLC

LEARNING OBJECTIVES

At the completion of this section, the learner will be able to do the following:

1. List three important questions to ask the mother in the prenatal period.
2. Assess the prenatal client's nipples and breasts for abnormalities that might interfere with function.
3. Identify types of nipple protractability, offering suggestions for prenatal and postpartum management of retracted or inverted nipples.
4. Instruct the prenatal and postpartum breastfeeding mother on proper nipple and breast care.

OUTLINE

V. Nipple and Areolar Assessment

    A. Nipple and areolar tissue

    B. Anatomical variations in nipples and breast

    C. Nipple assessment

VI. Correcting Nipple Problems

    A. Devices and techniques

    B. Treatment measures

VII. Nipple and Breast Care

PRE-TEST

For questions 1 to 4, choose the best answer.

1. Breastfeeding is more difficult for modern women because

    A. they are too nervous.
    B. most men prefer women not to breastfeed.
    C. financial pressures require employment outside the home.
    D. practical knowledge of breastfeeding management is not commonly known.

2. The content of breastfeeding education materials given in the prenatal period should include

    A. information on sore nipples and mastitis.
    B. information on how to supplement with formula.
    C. information that is accurate, uncomplicated, and specific to the client's needs.
    D. descriptions of treatment options for severe engorgement.

3. Counseling approaches for the prenatal period should emphasize

    A. advantages of breastfeeding over feeding manufactured milk.
    B. resolution of breastfeeding problems.
    C. dispelling misconceptions about breastfeeding held by the mother that influence the feeding decision.
    D. feeding frequency and feeding duration.

4. Milk-storage capacity

    A. is a fixed constant and does not vary from woman to woman.
    B. negatively impacts on lactation.
    C. may influence the baby's frequency and duration of feedings.
    D. can be enhanced by improving maternal diet.

For questions 5 to 8, choose the best answer from the following key:

    A. Inelastic breast tissue   **D. Galactorrhea**
    B. Elastic breast tissue   **E. Aplasia**
    C. Hypoplasia

5. Lactation is not possible.

6. A tendency to engorgement may be seen.

7. Continuous secretion of milk.

8. Underdevelopment of breast tissue.

For questions 9 to 13, choose the best answer from the following key:

    A. True   **B. False**

9. Retained placental fragments do not affect the establishment of lactation.

10. An anatomic cause of lactational insufficiency is Sheehan's syndrome.

11. In most women, the right breast is slightly larger than the left.

12. Smooth muscles in the nipple contract when stimulated to cause nipple erection.

13. Nipple length at rest is an important indication of protractability.

For questions 14 to 20, choose the best answer.

14. No special nipple interventions are needed for women with nipples that
    A. protract.
    B. retract.
    C. invert.
    D. dimple.

15. A _____ may be useful for correcting nipple problems prenatally.
    A. nipple sandwich
    B. nipple shield
    C. breast shell
    D. breast cream

16. Treatment measures for women with moderate-to-severe nipple retraction or complete nipple inversion include all of the following except:
    A. breastfeeding in the first two hours after birth.
    B. using corrective devices like breast shells prior to delivery.
    C. using the nipple sandwich technique for latching the baby onto the breast.
    D. using a towel to buff and toughen the nipple.

17. When teaching the patient prenatal nipple assessment, have the patient follow these steps:
    A. Patient removes her bra, stimulates her nipple with massage and/or stroking, and then applies the pinch test to see if the nipple will protrude.
    B. Patient removes her bra and after 10 minutes measures the diameter of the nipple.
    C. Patient is taught proper use of the breast pump and is instructed to use it to pull out nipples, then measures the difference in length.
    D. Patient wears breast shells for 24 hours in bra, then measures diameter of nipple.

18. The following terms describe the classifications of nipple protractability:
    A. protraction, retraction, inversion
    B. protraction, inversion, dimpling
    C. dimpling, inversion, retraction
    D. protraction, dimpling, retraction

19. Prenatal breast preparation includes
    A. removal of excess skin and debris from nipples, massaging the lateral sides of the breast, and pumping.
    B. breast massage, nipple buffing, and going without a bra.
    C. cleansing the areola with alcohol, wearing nipple shields and a good bra.
    D. washing the breast and nipples with plain water, using corrective devices when necessary, wearing a roomy bra.

20. Nursing bras are to be purchased
    A. while engorged.
    B. two weeks before the due date.
    C. five months prenatally.
    D. after engorgement subsides, approximately one week to two weeks postpartum.

Introduction

Breastfeeding is an art—a woman builds a repertoire of skills and techniques while feeding her infant. Women throughout human history have experienced breastfeeding in the course of their everyday lives. From early childhood, they learned the mannerisms and womanly habits through observing and pretending.

For modern women in many countries, breastfeeding is not part of the cultural norm. It is a topic discussed within private circles or associations. Choosing to breastfeed requires a woman to evaluate her personal feelings about modesty, the use of her body to feed her infant, her place in the social environment, and the opinions of family members. In addition, practical knowledge of breastfeeding management is not commonly known, with many women lacking breastfeeding role models.

For women who choose to breastfeed, it is a good idea for them to become informed about breastfeeding and its management to assure greater success and satisfaction. In the past 40 years, there has been increasing media coverage of breastfeeding. Bookstores have a wide selection of publications on breastfeeding. Other methods of preparation for breastfeeding include attending prenatal breast-feeding classes, observing a friend or relative breastfeed, and discussing breast-feeding with a knowledgeable health-care provider. In this way, the mother can focus on preparing her mind for the breastfeeding experience.

Prenatal Breastfeeding Education

PRENATAL CLASSES

Breastfeeding classes for expectant mothers are much like learning to drive a car on a computer simulator. One gains instruction and visual familiarity, but the experience is without the stimulation of actually driving a real car under ordinary conditions. Attending prenatal classes, however, means a mother-to-be is better prepared to approach the new experience. The following topics commonly are included in prenatal breastfeeding classes:

1. Breastfeeding importance
2. Breast anatomy and lactation physiology
3. Milk composition
4. Care of breasts and nipples
5. How to initiate breastfeeding
6. Management of breastfeeding
7. Self-assessment
8. Where to find support groups or help when needed
9. Reading and resource lists

Prenatal classes offer a private setting to encourage expectant mothers/couples to vocalize their concerns and fears and to ask questions. These classes are often facilitated by hospitals and clinics and taught by nurses, nutritionists, or lactation consultants. The scope and depth of the material varies from class to class (see Table 1A–1). Mothers should be advised to enrich their knowledge with reputable reading material known for its up-to-date accuracy and thorough information. In choosing client-education materials, the counselor should evaluate the content and presentation of the material. The content should be accurate, up-to-date, uncomplicated, and specific to the client and family's needs. The visuals should be consistent with the narrative and avoid emphasis on potential complications. The presentation should be organized for scanning with bold headings, short paragraphs, generous use of white space, and visuals that depict families similar to the target audience. The appropriateness of the reading level and length should be assessed (Bocar & Shrago, 1993).

There are often hidden messages in breastfeeding materials produced by formula companies. Breastfeeding is depicted as complicated, uncomfortable, immodest, and inconvenient. Implications are made that weaning after a few weeks or months is beneficial; and formula products, bottles, and nipples are promoted under the pretext of discussing weaning.

A benefit of attending a class is that a relationship develops between the student and the instructor that may be important to the breastfeeding mother when she needs encouragement and assistance. When prenatal classes include participants who are ambivalent about the infant-feeding decision, the instructor may choose to use a simple survey tool like the one in Figure 1A–1 to determine areas of misconceptions or lack of knowledge in the mothers. Then the class can be tailored to address the reasons a mother may not consider breastfeeding an option. Presenting both the advantages of breastfeeding and the hazards of artificial feeding will give the woman or couple the information needed to make an informed decision.

Table 1A-1   Sample Content for "How To" Breastfeeding Class

"Good Start Breastfeeding"

- Importance of early breastfeeding
  1. Frequent breastfeeding
  2. Rooming-in
     a. Learn early hunger cues
     b. Practice infant care skills
     c. Increase confidence

- Optimal infant state
  1. Comforting/consoling techniques
  2. Alerting techniques

- Avoid overuse of
  1. Swaddling and pacifiers

- Positioning and latch-on
  1. Discuss with visuals, video demonstration, demonstrate with doll
  2. Mother to return demonstrate

- What mother should notice
  1. Infant swallowing
  2. No sharp pain or severe discomfort

- Milk supply
  1. Milk removal principle of milk production; importance of colostrum
  2. Engorgement
     a. What and when to expect
     b. Prevention of severe engorgement
     c. Treatment and comfort measures
     d. Resolution does not mean lost milk supply
  3. Reassurance of adequacy of milk supply
     a. "How do I know if my baby is getting enough milk?"
  4. Nipple tenderness and engorgement
     a. What to expect
     b. Comfort measures
  5. Mother's lifestyle
     a. Nutrition
     b. Medications
        1. Recreational drugs, alcohol, nicotine
     c. If mother gets a cold
  6. Family life with baby
     a. Enjoying baby
     b. Fear of spoiling
     c. Family involvement
     d. Realistic expectations
     e. Withholding judgment about breastfeeding for two weeks

- What to expect during delivery

- When to seek assistance

Source: Bocar, DL (1993). *Breastfeeding Educator Program*, p. 115. Reprinted with permission of Lactation Consultant Services, Oklahoma City, OK.

Figure 1A-1

Breastfeeding Promotion Project Prenatal Survey Tool

Source: Adapted by East Central Health District Women, Infants and Children program from the Tennessee State Department of Health WIC program (1993).

1. PRENATAL INFANT FEEDING INTERVIEW

A. Today's Date _____ Chart Number _____

   Birthdate _____ Age _____ Name _____

   WIC _____ Prenatal _____ EDD _____ Address _____

B. How likely is it that you will breastfeed? _____

   1 = very likely   2 = somewhat likely   3 = don't know   4 = somewhat unlikely
   5 = very unlikely

   How long? _____ (Skip, if answer is 3, 4, or 5)

Please circle: A – Agree   D – Disagree   NS – Not Sure

	Agree	Disagree	Not Sure
1. Breastfeeding can help you lose weight.	A	D	NS
2. You can breastfeed in public without being obvious.	A	D	NS
3. You can breastfeed and bottle feed your baby in the same day.	A	D	NS
4. It is easier to bottle feed than to breastfeed.	A	D	NS
5. Formula is as good as breastmilk for your baby.	A	D	NS
6. You can go back to work or school and still breastfeed.	A	D	NS
7. Breastfeeding ties you down.	A	D	NS
8. Breastfeeding will make your breasts sag.	A	D	NS
9. Breastfeeding can help you feel closer to baby.	A	D	NS
10. Many women may not be able to make enough milk.	A	D	NS
11. Breastmilk can help protect baby against illness.	A	D	NS
12. Breastfeeding is painful.	A	D	NS
13. If you breastfeed, you cannot eat certain foods.	A	D	NS
14. You like the idea of breastfeeding.	A	D	NS

15. Some other reasons why women might feel uncomfortable about breastfeeding. Are these some reasons that you think might be important to you?
    ☐ size of my breast   ☐ smoking   ☐ birth control pill   ☐ other _____

INDIVIDUAL COUNSELING

Survey tools can be effective in individual counseling sessions as well. They allow the counselor to quickly identify how to direct the counseling. If a client or patient knows breastfeeding is far superior to artificial baby milk, then a discussion of breastfeeding advantages may miss the point. If the same mother identified on the survey a concern over her diet, smoking habits, etc., the counselor would be more effective by recognizing her concerns, empathizing with her, and presenting information to her on how her lifestyle can fit with breastfeeding. Presenting the information in a counseling style that shows empathy, recognizes patient concerns, and keeps the patient involved in the counseling process is more effective. See Module 1, *The Support of Breastfeeding,* Chapter 1, for more on the barriers to breastfeeding and counseling approaches that work to increase incidence, exclusivity, and duration of breastfeeding.

PEER SUPPORT

Another source of information for the expectant mother is a friend or relative who has breastfed successfully or is breastfeeding. Observing infants go to the breast and feed at the breast can greatly enhance a woman's self-confidence in her ability to breastfeed. Seeing someone close to her engage in breastfeeding gives the mother an opportunity to ask specific questions related to feeding a baby at the breast and will help alleviate any fears she may have of whether she is "doing it right." The peer concept has been very successful, as evidenced by La Leche League International's growth. Peer leaders, resource mothers, etc., have also emerged as supportive personnel in the breastfeeding promotion programs of the Special Supplemental Nutrition Program for Women, Infants and Children (WIC) in the United States.

Prenatal Breast Assessment

Prenatal breast assessment should be provided for every woman preparing to breastfeed. The assessment can be performed by the nurse, lactation consultant, public health worker, or physician. Breasts come in various sizes and shapes. Descriptions, such as flat, upright, nonlactating, firm, engorged, rounded, saggy, empty, full, are often used. The size, symmetry, and shape of a woman's breast have little to do with her ability to lactate successfully. It is the glandular tissue of the breast that produces and secretes milk, not the fatty tissue.

MILK-STORAGE CAPACITY

Research does indicate that there is a great variation in the milk-storage capacity among women (Daly, Owens, & Hartman, 1993). Women with smaller breasts may have less glandular storage tissue and less area in the ducts and lactiferous sinuses for milk. Milk production in a 24-hour period is reported to range between 450 g per day and 1200 g per day, with a mean of 750 to 800 g per day (Institute of Medicine, 1991). A mother with less storage capacity may or may not have to offer more frequent feeding to meet the infant's needs. If a woman with a smaller area for milk storage has an infant that requires less than the norm of milk to grow steadily and thrive, one may not see very frequent feedings. The same mother may have another child who is a robust and vigorous eater and requires calories at the upper limit of the norm; feeding more frequently compensates for the lower-than-average volume at any one feed. The point is we should not dwell on the size of the breast; but rather help the mother and family understand the design of the system, emphasizing the infant's role in controlling the feedings.

BREAST TEXTURE AND SHAPE

Breast texture can be assessed by palpation. Inelastic breast tissue has firm, taut skin and cannot be picked up easily. Inelastic breast tissue is more prone to engorgement and is reported to benefit from prenatal massaging and engorgement prevention (Lawrence, 1989). Elastic breast tissue is looser, and the overlying skin is picked up easily.

During an early prenatal visit, the health-care provider should do a breast examination to determine if any corrective treatments are needed to further prepare the expectant mother for breastfeeding. Familiarity with variations in nipples and breast shapes (see Figure 1A–2) assists the counselor in offering guidance to mothers who may require modification of some of the latch-on and positioning techniques due to individual body-type variations.

The prenatal counselor should also question the mother-to-be about her medical condition, medication use, and any previous breastfeeding experience(s) as a screen for those mothers who would benefit from additional prenatal counseling.

Figure 1A–2

Breasts come in all sizes and shapes

Source: Diane Davis, artist. Concept from Susan Aldridge, artist for Huggins, K (1990). *The Nursing Mother's Companion*, p. 26. Boston: Harvard Common Press. Reprinted with permission.

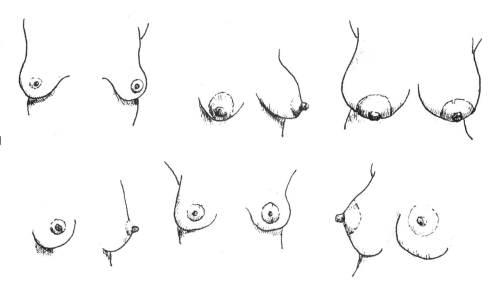

Assessment Questions to Ask the Mother

1. Did the breast increase in size during pregnancy?—The alveoli and ducts proliferate in pregnancy, causing an increase in the glandular tissue and thus the increased size of the breast.

2. Is there a history of fibrocystic breast disease, cancer, augmentation or reduction surgery, etc.?—Procedures that alter the breast should be discussed to determine if glandular and/or nervous tissue may have been damaged or severed.

3. If the mother has breastfed previously, inquire about any breast problems, such as mastitis, pathologic engorgement, galactoceles, sore nipples, etc.—Breast problems can often be prevented with appropriate management. The counselor should be aware of previous problems in order to provide the appropriate preventive counseling.

4. What medication, prescriptive or over the counter, does the mother take on a regular basis?—While the majority of medications will not interfere with lactation, there are some that do. See Module 4, *The Management of Breastfeeding*, Chapter 2.

5. If she discontinued breastfeeding prior to her personal goal, ask why to determine if it was because of a perceived milk insufficiency.—Mothers often discontinue breastfeeding because they think they do not have enough milk. In fact, the mother's milk supply may have been adequate. Frequent feedings and infant behavior during appetite spurts may be misinterpreted by the mother as an indication her milk supply is low.

6. Are there any breast abnormalities that may affect lactation?—See the next section.

Breast Abnormalities

Osborne (1991) describes a wide range of breast abnormalities:

1. Unilateral hypoplasia, normal contralateral
2. Bilateral hypoplasia with asymmetry
3. Unilateral hyperplasia, normal contralateral
4. Bilateral hyperplasia with asymmetry
5. Unilateral hypoplasia, contralateral hypoplasia
6. Unilateral hypoplasia of breast, thorax, and pectoral muscles (Poland's syndrome)

More information on some of these specific breast abnormalities follows.

Agalactia—Absence of milk secretion after childbirth.

Amastia—Absence of glandular tissue, areola, and nipples. Lactation is not possible.

Anisomastia—Term used to describe significant size difference between two breasts.

Aplasia—Absence of glandular tissue. Areola and nipple are present. Lactation is not possible.

Athelia—Absence of areola and nipple. Rare in the presence of a normal breast. Most often observed with hypoplasia. Milk production occurs but no delivery possible. Severe engorgement results, and lactation is not possible.

Galactorrhea—Continuous secretion of milk from the breast after the cessation of nursing or the spontaneous secretion of milk from the breast under nonphysiological conditions. Drugs such as reserpine, methyldopa, and phenothiazines have been reported to cause abnormal milk secretion. Galactorrhea may be a symptom of hyperprolactinemia, although only 30% of women with this condition are reported to have higher than normal prolactin levels (Frantz, Kleinberg, & Noel, 1972). Sensitivity to normal circulating prolactin levels may account for these women's sensitivity (Friesen & Cowden, 1989). Intrauterine devices with copper also have been reported to cause abnormal milk secretion (Horne & Scott, 1969). Central nervous system lesions, chest wall lesions, and medical conditions (Cushing's disease, hepatic cirrhosis, hypothyroidism, sarcoidosis, chronic renal failure, Hand–Schuller–Christian disease) can also cause galactorrhea.

Hyperadenia—Presence of mammary tissue without nipples. This has been reported to occur in the right axillary Tail of Spence and to be separated from the rest of the glandular tissue. Plastic surgeons may remove the tissue if the woman desires to lactate because the area can produce pain from the secretion of milk without an appropriate nipple; swelling may be pronounced and the potential for mastitis may be increased.

Hypermastia—Presence of accessory mammary glands, which are remnants of the embryonic stage. These accessory mammary glands, called the supernumary nipples, are found along the mammary ridge, from the clavicular to inguinal regions. There may also be glandular tissue without nipple/areolar tissue. Synonymous with polymastia.

Hyperplasia—Overdevelopment of the fatty breast tissue.

Hyperthelia—Presence of nipple tissue without mammary gland tissue.

Hypoplasia—Underdevelopment of breast tissue. In severe hypoplasia, it takes pregnancy to indicate whether there is a complete lack of breast tissue. Synonymous with micromastia in that both refer to underdevelopment of breast tissue, but hypoplasia is a secondary developmental disorder (see Table 1A–2). In many cases, lactation is possible.

Megaareola—Enlargement of areolar tissue, often referred to as "puffy" areola. Normal lactation is possible.

Micromastia—Micromastia is synonymous with hypoplasia in that both refer to underdevelopment of breast tissue. Micromastia is a primary developmental disorder (see Table 1A–2) and may result in lactation insufficiency.

Microthelia—Underdeveloped nipple and areolar tissue. There may be minimal milk delivery, and breastfeeding may be difficult or not possible.

Polygalactia—Excessive secretion or flow of milk.

Polymastia—Presence of accessory mammary glandular tissue and/or breasts. Often the accessory tissue lacks the areola and nipple, but sometimes it may have areolar and nipple tissue (supernumary nipples).

Table 1A–2   Primary and Secondary Developmental Disorders

PRIMARY DEVELOPMENTAL DISORDERS

- Poland's syndrome
- Amastia
- Mammary aplasia
- Micromastia
- Athelia
- Polymastia

SECONDARY DEVELOPMENTAL DISORDERS

- Hypoplasia
- Microthelia
- Megaareola
- Macrothelia
- Juvenile mammary hyperplasia
- Gestational mammary hypertrophy

Source: Craig, HR (1993). *Lactational Insufficiency and Induced Lactation.* Lecture presented at International Lactation Consultants Association annual meeting, Scottsdale, AZ. Reprinted with permission.

Trunk Breast/Macrothelia—An unusual type of malformation characterized by areola enlargement and herniation of the anterior parenchyma, which causes the areola to stick straight out or hang down from the residual breast. Latching may be difficult or not possible.

In addition to the preceding anatomic causes of lactational insufficiency, there are endocrine, physiologic, pregnancy-related, systemic, and idiopathic causes of lactational insufficiency (see Table 1A–3). These are discussed in Module 3, *The Science of Breastfeeding*, Chapter 1.

Table 1A–3 Causes of Lactational Insufficiency

Categories	Signs of Abnormality	Common Terms
Anatomic	Abnormal breast development or anatomy	Amastia Mammary aplasia Micromastia Athelia Microthelia Hypertrophic dystocia
Endocrine Central	Hypothalamic abnormality or dysfunction, pituitary gland insufficiency	Kallman's syndrome Low prolactin production or release
Peripheral	Systemic hormone abnormality	Hypothyroid Hyperandrogenism High postpartum estrogen levels
Acquired	Injury to lactation-related gland	Sheehan's syndrome
Physiologic	Abnormal or absent breast tissue response to normal hormone levels	Prolactin receptor deficiency Prolactin receptor dysfunction Steroid receptor deficiency
Pregnancy-related	Inappropriate placental hormone production	Retained placental fragments Low placental lactogen
Systemic	Disorders involving the entire body	Dehydration Poor nutrition Stress
Idiopathic	Unknown causes	Unknown causes

Source: Craig, HR (1993). *Lactational Insufficiency and Induced Lactation.* Lecture presented at International Lactation Consultants Association annual meeting, Scottsdale, AZ. Reprinted with permission.

Nipple and Areolar Assessment

NIPPLE AND AREOLAR TISSUE

The mammary papillae or *nipple* is found at the center of each breast, usually at the fourth intercostal space. The *areola* is a specialized, pigmented skin surrounding the nipple.

During lactation, the nipple areola averages 6.4 cm in diameter, the erectile portion of the nipple averages 1.6 cm in diameter, and the erectile nipple length averages 0.7 cm (Ziemer & Pigeon, 1993). Both contain smooth erectile muscles that contract when stimulated to make the nipple erect. The muscles also function as a closing mechanism for the 15 to 25 lactiferous ducts that are embedded in connective tissue as they merge to end as small orifices within the nipple. The areola contains openings for apocrine glands, which hypertrophy in pregnancy and are called Montgomery's tubercles or follicles. These sebaceouslike glands secrete fatty acids (sebum), which lowers the pH, thereby possibly serving as antiseptic agents. The structural elements of areolar and nipple tissue are reviewed in Module 3, *The Science of Breastfeeding*, Chapter 1; and the principles of wound healing specific to the areola and nipple are reviewed in Chapter 2 in this module.

ANATOMICAL VARIATIONS IN NIPPLES AND BREASTS

There are many breast/areola/nipple combinations: large breasts, small areola, small nipple; small breasts, large areola, small nipple; medium breasts, small areola, large nipple, etc. (see Table 1A–4). Recommendations that the infant should take the complete areola into the mouth are misleading. It might better be stated than the infant should take as much of the areolar tissue in as his mouth allows. Women with large breasts usually do need to support their breast during the entire feeding in the early weeks to keep the weight of the underside of the breast off the infant's chin. Small-breasted women may not need to provide breast support but may find, in the early days of initiating feedings, support of the breast gives them more control as they work to quickly center the nipple and pull the infant onto the breast when the infant's mouth is opened.

Table 1A–4   Size of Areola and Diameter of Nipple

Size of Areola	Diameter of Nipple
Small – ½"–¾"	Small – ¼"
Medium – 1"	Medium – ⅜"
Large – 1"–1½"	Large – ½"
Ex. Large – 2"	Ex. Large – ¾"

Source: Marmet, C, Shell, E (1986). *Lactation Forms: A Guide to Lactation Consultant Charting.* Reprinted with permission of the Lactation Institute, Encino, CA (818/955-1913).

In most women, the left breast is slightly larger than the right. Striking asymmetry may mean inadequate glandular tissue; but this is rare, and the presence of striking asymmetry does not prevent the mother from breastfeeding her infant(s), although additional supplementation may be necessary (Neifert & Seacat, 1986).

NIPPLE ASSESSMENT

The length of the resting nipple is not important because the infant forms the areola tissue and nipple into a teat. What is important is the nipple graspability and protractability (see Figure 1A–3). The appearance of the nipple in its resting state is not as important as how the nipple responds when the areolar tissue is compressed between the infant's gums. A quick and easy method that can be performed at the beginning of the third trimester to check for function of the nipple is the pinch test. The nipple-pinch test is used to determine the protractability, or lack thereof, and should be performed during the prenatal breast assessment. Sometimes a nipple may not appear everted on visual inspection, but it functions fine when the infant goes to breast.

Accurate nipple assessment involves

1. having the breasts free from compression. After bra removal, allow the skin time to relax.
2. observing the nipple diameter and height at rest.
3. observing the nipple when stimulated via massage or stroking by the mother.
4. pressing the areola on both sides of the nipple to determine protractability. The mother or caregiver places the thumb and forefinger on either side behind the nipple. She should gently compress the fingers together so as to protract the nipple and areola to form a teat. If the nipple everts out easily, it is protractile.

Inversion of the nipple is a problem if it interferes with the infant's latching on to the breast. It is believed to be caused by adhesions (bands of connective tissue) at the base of the nipple, which hold the skin to the underlying tissue. During the third trimester of pregnancy, the skin becomes more elastic in response to hormones; but some of the cells may remain attached. During vigorous nursing, if these cells do not break loose, a whole layer of tissue may lift up, which causes blisters and cracks. In lay and professional publications, the adhered nipple is sometimes referred to as flat, inverted, dimpled, or folded.

Nipple function has been classified into three states: protraction, retraction, and inversion (Riordan & Auerbach, 1993). *Protraction* refers to the normal functional response of the nipple—moving forward when stimulated. *Retraction* is when the nipple moves inward in response to stimulation; it can be minimal or moderate-to-severe. Minimal retraction may not require intervention if the infant's suck is strong enough to exert sufficient pressure to pull the nipple forward. It may cause difficulties for the premature infant or infant with a weak suck. Moderate-to-severe retraction involves a nipple that retracts to a level even with or behind the surrounding areola when stimulated. Intervention to stretch the nipple outward may improve protractility. *Inversion* is when all or part of the nipple is drawn

Figure 1A–3

Protractability

Source: King, FS (1992). *Help-ing Mothers to Breastfeed,* Revised Edition, p. 52. Nairobi, Kenya: African Medical and Research Foundation (AMRF). Reprinted with permission.

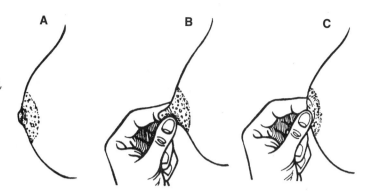

Occasionally a nipple really does not protract well. If you try to pull it out, it goes deeper into the breast. Protractability is more important than the length of a nipple.

A. A short nipple. Is it protractile or not?
B. If you can pull it out like this, then it protracts well.
C. If it goes in like this when you try to pull it out, then it is not protractile.

inward within the folds of the areola. Simple inversion indicates the nipple moves outward to protraction with manual pressure or cold stimuli (pseudo-inversion). Complete inversion is when the nipple does not respond to manual or cold pressure because adhesions bind the nipple inward or, in rare cases, when there is a congenital absence of the nipple. See Chapter 2, Section C in this module for a description of nipple classification with information on management strategies.

Correcting Nipple Problems

Three devices and one technique to correct nipple problems have been described: breast shells, dimple rings, and modified disposable syringes; and Hoffman's exercises. See Chapter 2, Section C in this module for drawings of these devices and management techniques for the mother having difficulties with breastfeeding due to nipple problems. The nipple sandwich technique was developed to assist with latch-on for the mother with retracted or inverted nipples and while used after birth is mentioned in this prenatal section.

DEVICES AND TECHNIQUES

1. *Breast shells*—Do not confuse breast shells with nipple shields. Breast shells are made of nonmalleable plastic, with two parts that are worn over the areola/nipple area inside the bra of the woman with moderate-to-severe nipple retraction or complete nipple inversion. The back portion of the breast shell has a small concentric opening that fits around the base of the nipple where it joins the areolar tissue. The breast shell works by applying pressure to stretch the adhesions that keep the teat from protracting. The front portion may have air vents. Some are packaged with a cylinder-shaped piece of gauze to be placed in the breast shell to collect leakage. If used, these should be changed frequently. Recently, the efficacy of breast shells has been questioned (Alexander et al., 1993).

2. *Marmet dimple ring*—The dimple ring is another device used for nipples that invert partially or dimple. It is used after feedings to allow sufficient air drying of the area of the nipple that dimples. It can also be worn prior to feedings to evert all parts of the nipple tissue.

3. *Modified disposable syringe*—An article published in the *Journal of Human Lactation* discussed a homemade device for drawing out an inverted nipple using a syringe (Kesaree et al., 1993). A commercial application of this concept is produced by Maternal Concepts; it is called Evert-It™.

4. *Hoffman's exercises*—This exercise is often taught to women with retracted, inverted, or dimpled nipples. Recent research has shown neither a positive or negative effect on nipple protractability using this technique (Alexander et al., 1993). The technique's benefit may come instead from the mother's handling of her breast, which may be important in the psychological preparation for breastfeeding.

   The technique for Hoffman's exercises is easy: The mother places her thumbs on each side of the base of the nipple, where it meets the areola. Then the mother presses in firmly against the breast tissue and at the same time pulls the thumbs away from each other. The technique may bruise the nipples if done incorrectly and cause uterine contractions by stimulating oxytocin release.

5. *Nipple sandwich*—This technique for handling and offering the breast to ease latch-on difficulties was developed by Barbara Heiser, RN, IBCLC. It is included in this prenatal section with other ways to correct nipple problems; however, the nipple sandwich cannot be of use until after the baby arrives. The nipple sandwich is described in Section B, Feeding at the Breast.

TREATMENT MEASURES

The following treatment measures are for women with moderate-to-severe nipple retraction or complete nipple inversion:

1. Use corrective devices, such as breast shells, in their bras for several hours per day in the few months prior to delivery (last trimester). After delivery, they can also be worn a half-hour before nursing, if needed. Purchase or make a bra extender to keep the bra from binding when the shells are in place. Wash and sterilize the breast shells regularly. Recognize that this is an optional exercise until more research on its efficacy is available.
2. Practice Hoffman's exercises several times daily if there is no history of preterm labor.
3. Breastfeed in the first hour after birth.
4. Give no artificial nipples or teats to the baby.
5. Stimulate the nipple to stand out by using a hospital electric pump, practicing nipple rolling, applying ice, or using a disposable syringe to evert the nipple.
6. Wear breast shells for a half-hour before nursing, if engorged.
7. If engorged, manually express milk to soften the areola before nursing.
8. To assist latch-on by the baby, position the thumb above the areola and fingers below; and push the breast to the chest wall, forming a nipple sandwich.
9. In extreme cases, the use of a nipple shield may be necessary. The nipple shield should be regarded as a last resort and is not without risks. See Chapter 2 in this module for instructions on the appropriate and correct use of the nipple shield.

Nipple and Breast Care

Older literature on breastfeeding instructed mothers to engage in harsh methods in order to be ready for breastfeeding. Current information has revealed a clearer understanding. Nipples do not require buffing with a towel or brush to "toughen" the skin for nursing. Nor do breasts need manual expression in the prenatal period to assure generous milk supply. Such rigorous measures as buffing remove the epithelial cells from nipple tissue, exposing the skin to the risk of infection and cracking. Breast stimulation may induce labor; therefore, expression of colostrum before birth may predispose a mother to premature labor. Correct nipple and breast care creates minimal stimulation and no trauma to skin tissue.

The woman should be instructed to care for her nipples and breasts in the following ways:

1. Wash with plain water. Avoid the use of soaps, alcohol, or astringents on breasts or nipples. Otherwise, natural emollients secreted by the Montgomery's tubercles could be removed.
2. Wear corrective devices to improve nipple protractability and/or do Hoffman's exercises.
3. Choose a comfortable, easy-to-manage nursing bra that offers support without binding. Advise the mother that if she purchases nursing bras during the last two weeks of pregnancy, they need to be larger than her current breast size. Encourage the mother to wait until approximately a week after delivery to be fitted for her nursing bras.
4. For dry skin types, massage a teardrop amount of a natural emollient, such as anhydrous, low-residue, low-detergent lanolin into nipple folds to increase elasticity and internal moisture of the skin.

The combination of preparing the mind to breastfeed and lining up support for the early postpartum period will more than prepare the average woman for breastfeeding. For those women in whom a prenatal breast and nipple/areolar tissue assessment reveals a potential problem, such as retracted or inverted nipples, the simple devices and techniques described above may be helpful.

POST-TEST

For questions 1 to 4, choose the best answer.

1. In countries where breastfeeding is not the cultural norm, women
   A. may be influenced not to breastfeed by family members and friends.
   B. can be negatively influenced to breastfeed by discussing breastfeeding in prenatal classes.
   C. may not be worried over breastfeeding in public.
   D. know the hazards of manufactured milk feeding.

2. When choosing education materials for prenatal clients, be sure to
   A. include pamphlets on sore nipples, engorgement, and mastitis.
   B. ask formula companies for free literature.
   C. select materials with visuals that emphasize problem resolution.
   D. select material that is on the client's reading level and depicts culturally similar families in its visuals.

3. Counseling approaches that work in promoting breastfeeding include
   A. ones that primarily emphasize the advantages of breastfeeding.
   B. ones that show empathy and allow the client to verbalize concerns, fears, or misconceptions.
   C. showing audiovisuals of breastfeeding women resolving difficulties.
   D. outlining the rules for breastfeeding.

4. Observing an infant of a friend or relative feed at the breast can
   A. intimidate and scare first-time mothers.
   B. ease anxiety and increase self-confidence in the mother.
   C. keep mothers from asking questions about breastfeeding.
   D. cause a mother to reject breastfeeding as her method of infant feeding.

For questions 5 to 9, choose the best answer from the following key:
   A. Milk-storage capacity
   B. Breast changes during pregnancy
   C. Prolactin-receptor deficiency
   D. Sheehan's syndrome
   E. Retained placental fragments

5. Endocrine cause of lactational insufficiency.

6. Pregnancy-related cause of lactational insufficiency.

7. Varies greatly among women.

8. Physiologic cause of lactational insufficiency.

9. Due to proliferation of glandular tissue.

For questions 10 to 14, choose the best answer.

10. For the prenatal client, Hoffman's exercises may help when
    A. diagnosing nipple protractability.
    B. correcting nipple protractability.
    C. strengthening pelvic-floor muscles.
    D. all of the above.

11. In assessing the client's breasts and nipples in preparation for breastfeeding, observe the

    A. protractability of nipple.
    B. size of bra, color of nipple, and diameter of areola.
    C. width of breast, diameter of areola, and any skin discolorations.
    D. Montgomery's tubercules activity, nipple secretions, and weight of breasts.

12. Nipple corrective treatments should begin

    A. two hours after birth.
    B. before the first feed.
    C. six to twelve weeks before estimated date of confinement.
    D. only when nipples become traumatized.

13. Nipple erection is dependent upon

    A. the baby licking the nipple before latch-on.
    B. doing nipple rolling before each feed.
    C. the length of the nipple.
    D. the erection of smooth muscle when stimulated.

14. Which of the following holds is the best choice for the client with complete inversion?

    A. Scissors hold
    B. Nipple sandwich
    C. C-hold
    D. Dancer hand position

For questions 15 to 20, choose the best answer from the following key:

   A. True   B. False

15. During pregnancy, nipple toughening is necessary to prevent sore nipples.

16. Gaining knowledge prenatally about breastfeeding is important to breastfeeding success.

17. Nipples that fold over or dimple in at the tips are unsuitable for breastfeeding, thus indicating the mother should not attempt to breastfeed.

18. Mothers should be warned of problems with latch-on if they have complete nipple inversion on one or both breasts.

19. It is recommended that women purchase nursing bras prenatally.

20. Measuring the areolar and nipple diameter are ways to determine nipple protractability.

SECTION B

Feeding at the Breast

Rebecca F. Black, MS, RD/LD, IBCLC
Donna Calhoun, BS, IBCLC

LEARNING OBJECTIVES

At the completion of this section, the learner will be able to do the following:

1. List three signs of an infant's readiness to breastfeed.
2. List three signs of a mother's readiness to breastfeed.
3. Describe two techniques for supporting the breast while breastfeeding.
4. Instruct the client on breastfeeding basics, including positioning, cueing, and latching techniques.

OUTLINE

I. When the Baby Arrives

II. Assessing the Infant's Readiness to Breastfeed

    A. The responsive state of the infant

    B. Hunger cues

    C. Crying

    D. Calming techniques

    E. Reflexes of newborns

III. Assessing the Mother's Readiness to Breastfeed

    A. Physical and emotional comfort

    B. Psychosocial concerns of new parents

    C. Prefeeding activities

IV. Support of the Breast

    A. C-hold (palmar grasp)

    B. Scissors hold

    C. Nipple sandwich

V. Positioning

    A. Cradle or madonna hold

    B. Modified cradle hold

    C. Clutch hold

    D. Lying-down position

    E. Specialty positions

VI. Cueing and Latch-on Techniques

VII. Feeding Management

    A. Feeding duration

    B. Breastfeeding frequency

    C. Removing baby from the breast

PRE-TEST

For questions 1 to 6, choose the best answer.

1. Immediately after birth, most healthy, term infants exhibit

    A. subdued, placid behavior.

    B. alertness and rooting movements.

    C. symptoms of hypoglycemia.

    D. dangerously low body temperatures.

2. In providing care to new parents, try all of the following except

    A. offering several alternate choices for positioning.

    B. dividing tasks into easily mastered segments.

    C. providing consistent suggestions.

    D. expressing confidence in their abilities.

3. The responsive state of the infant is

    A. usually not evident until the second-day postpartum.

    B. during crying.

    C. a quiet alert state.

    D. after feedings.

4. Calming and consoling techniques include all of the following except

    A. placing a crying baby away from noise.

    B. physical security and tactile stimulation.

    C. soft, rhythmic sounds.

    D. gentle motion of carrying, rocking, swinging.

5. Prior to a breastfeed, the mother should

    A. clean her nipples.

    B. wash her hands.

    C. apply a nipple shield.

    D. pump her breasts.

6. Warm compresses, stroking and shaking the breast, and breast massage will

    A. reduce nipple soreness.

    B. cause vasoconstriction of the blood vessels in the breast.

    C. interfere with lactogenesis.

    D. help elicit the milk-ejection reflex.

For questions 7 to 9, choose the best answer from the following key:

    A. C-hold

    B. Scissors hold

    C. Nipple sandwich

7. May completely prevent baby from latching.

8. May be useful for retracted or inverted nipples.

9. Allows the mother to lift the weight of the breast off the baby's chin.

For questions 10 to 16, choose the best answer from the following key:

    A. Cradle- or madonna-hold position

    B. Modified cradle-hold position

    C. Clutch-hold position

    D. Lying-down position

10. Good for women with sore perineum.

11. Good for getting more rest during night feeds.

12. Good for small or premature baby.

13. Awkward for women with long limbs, slender bodies, and large babies.

14. May be more difficult than other holds when stabilization of the head is essential.

15. A sitting position good for women with inverted nipples.

16. Along with clutch hold, this hold is good for stabilization of the head.

For questions 17 to 20, choose the best answer.

17. Cueing the infant for latch-on involves

    A. positioning the infant so his or her cheek faces the nipple.

    B. pressing the infant's face very close to the breast.

    C. tickling the infant's lower lip and waiting for his or her mouth to open wide.

    D. grasping the infant by the head to turn him or her toward the nipple.

18. The health-care provider's role in assisting feeding at the breast includes

    A. assessing readiness; and assisting with positioning, cueing, and latching.

    B. bringing the infant to the mother and watching as she feeds the baby.

    C. telling the mother what she is doing wrong.

    D. checking on how long the infant fed.

19. Skin-to-skin contact facilitates all of the following except

   A. raising the infant's body temperature.
   B. colonizing the infant with the mother's flora.
   C. helping the infant learn his or her mother's smell.
   D. delaying the first feeding at the breast.

20. The first milk available for the baby is

   A. prelacteal milk.
   B. transitional milk.
   C. colostrum.
   D. mature milk.

When the Baby Arrives

Following birth, breastfeeding provides a natural reconnection between mother and infant. Hopefully, the first nursing occurs immediately or shortly after birth. While the volume of colostrum available is small, the infant can experiment with the nipple and learn to attach and suck correctly, thus eliciting the normal suck–swallow–breathe response. Breastfeeding, while not difficult, is complex and the small volume of colostrum allows the infant the opportunity to learn before the copious milk-ejection reflex occurs, which is often by the second- to third-day postpartum.

Colostrum is the ideal first food for the newborn. Colostrum helps the baby balance its system after the rigors of birth. Even if aspirated in the lungs, it will not create difficulty for the baby, because it is easily absorbed into the tissues. The importance of early feedings of colostrum on gastrointestinal and immune function is discussed in Module 3, *The Science of Breastfeeding*, Chapter 2.

The early postbirth hours are a critical period for the establishment of lactation. Complementing or supplementing the small amount of colostrum with extra fluids when this is not medically indicated is professional mismanagement and can alter the normal course of lactation. Research by Widstrom et al. (1987) validated the ability of infants from unmedicated deliveries to initiate spontaneous feeding behavior unassisted when placed in a prone position between their mother's breasts. In these infants, sucking and rooting movements began at a mean of 15 minutes, hand-to-mouth movements at 34 minutes, and spontaneous sucking at 55 minutes. These researchers were so amazed by what they saw that a video-tape of this spontaneous unassisted behavior was made. Viewing this video is humbling and raises the question of why so many infants have initial difficulty getting on the breast.

Many of the answers to this question lie in the birthing procedures and the proto-cols of early postpartum care that interrupt and/or prolong the placement of the infant to the breast. Because so many mothers and babies experience early difficulties, the health professional is often called on to assist the infant to breast.

Depending upon the events during the birth and medications taken by the mother for pain, a newborn will often be ready and eager to root and suck within minutes after birth. The mother's breasts are already prepared with colostrum to feed her baby, whether or not she has seen any evidence of prenatal leaking. A chain reaction of response triggers initiate bonding. When the baby is born and the effort of labor is diminished, mother and infant are at their peak of awareness and imprinting. Their first response is to get acquainted and actualize each other's presence. This is an intense and crucial moment, emotionally charged and difficult to duplicate again. The birth attendants and caregivers need to acknowledge its importance and allow the mother to be involved as much as she is physically able. Medical procedures are important and necessary; however, unless a problem warrants immediate action, it benefits the mother and newborn to have time to settle down and relax. Administrative agendas can usually be done in due time.

Attendants can be most helpful by allowing the mother and baby to nurse skin-to-skin on the birthing bed or table, even after a cesarean birth. Using a blanket to keep mother and baby warm is sufficient to maintain body temperatures. Work in preterm infants has revealed that in skin-to-skin contact the infant's needs regulate the mother's body temperature (Anderson, 1991). Infants have a well-developed sense of smell and skin-to-skin contact helps the infant to recognize the mother's smell. The infant's skin is colonized with the mother's normal flora in skin-to-skin contact, and mothers have been reported to recognize their infants by touch after one hour of contact with the infant (Kaitz et al., 1992).

Birthing women consider open communication with caregivers highly important. They want to know they can trust the people and policies during their stay; therefore, it is essential for the caregiver to be an attentive and thoughtful listener. Every birthing mother planning to breastfeed expects the staff caring for her to be knowledgeable about breastfeeding management and how to get the baby latched on to the breast. Mothers become confused and frustrated when faced with caregivers who are inconsistent with instructions and methodology. Such inconsistency places the mother and infant in a poor position to begin breastfeeding and at risk for ensuing problems after discharge. Many hospitals and clinics around the world are implementing breastfeeding task forces or designating members of staff to be responsible for evaluating current standard procedures for breastfeeding management and recommending needed changes. See Module 1, *The Support of Breastfeeding*, Chapter 3 for information on optimal birthing policies for breastfeeding. The focus here is on the process of breastfeeding itself.

The first feeding triggers an imprinting mechanism in the baby. If presented with a bottle for the first feed, the infant will develop tongue and jaw adaptations for using a gravity-fed device. Techniques to "bring down" or "call up" the mother's milk are eliminated because the bottle requires no priming to work. Thus, there is no incentive to work for a feed. Continued use of the bottle during the transitional period can lead to "nipple confusion," in which the baby will not accept the breast. Nipple confusion is discussed and treatment measures suggested in Chapter 2 in this module.

By offering the breast immediately after birth, the baby becomes accustomed to using his senses to locate the breast and to feed. The infant becomes adapted to the mother's soft skin, molding the breast tissue to his mouth, and using the entire jaw and tongue to suck.

Assessing the Infant's Readiness to Breastfeed

THE RESPONSIVE STATE OF THE INFANT

The responsive state is ideally a quiet, alert state. The infant is in an alert and eager state from birth to two hours. The infant falls into a light to deep sleep between the second and twentieth (plus) hours. Increasing wakefulness characterizes the infant from 20 to 24 hours with a cluster of 5 to 10 feeding episodes over two to three hours followed by a four- to five-hour deep sleep (Riordan & Auerbach, 1993). By initiating the first feed soon after delivery, nature takes care of mother and baby. The sucking response is most intense during the first hour after birth. Delaying gratification has been reported to make it more difficult for the baby to learn to suck later (Anderson et al., 1982; Eppink, 1969). Uterine contractions are stimulated by sucking, which aids in placental expulsion and helps control maternal blood loss. The infant quickly begins to receive the immunologic advantage of colostrum, and the infant's digestive peristalsis and gut maturation is stimulated.

HUNGER CUES

In the responsive state, the infant displays the following early hunger cues:

- Rooting
- Mouth opening
- Lip licking, placing hand in mouth
- Sucking and/or chewing on hands or fingers
- Flexion of arms
- Clenching of fists
- Motor activity

When the mother and baby are kept together after birth, the mother can be taught to recognize early hunger cues in her infant.

CRYING

Crying is a late hunger cue, and it is best to offer the breast before crying begins. Frantic crying will increase latch-on difficulty. Crying is not without bad effects in the infant. It obstructs venous return in the inferior vena cava, reestablishing fetal circulation. Hypoxemia occurs with reestablished fetal circulation. Crying also obstructs venous return in the superior vena cava, increasing cerebral blood volume and decreasing cerebral oxygenation in a fluctuating pattern. Fluctuating patterns of cerebral blood flow are associated with intracranial hemorrhage. Since crying is not innocuous, every effort should be made to minimize it. The family can be shown the infant's subtle cues and communication signals. The mother can be assisted to identify early hunger signals.

CALMING TECHNIQUES

Crying and fussy babies should be calmed prior to offering the breast. Some general guidelines to consoling an infant include responding quickly, keeping the infant warm, encouraging flexion of the infant's body and physical security through swaddling and holding the infant snugly, and carrying the infant. Infants may need interaction and stimulation to distract them from the cause of discomfort. Parents report car rides and placing the infant in an infant seat on top of the clothes dryer often console a fussy baby. (See Table 1B–1.)

Table 1B–1   Calming and Consoling Techniques

- Kinesthetic Stimulation
  1. Holding
     a. Gentle motion in all three planes (amount of motion similar to intrauterine motion)
        1) Side to side
        2) Up and down
        3) Front to back
     b. Carry, rock, swing, gently bounce

- Tactile Stimulation
  1. Skin-to-skin contact
  2. Massaging
  3. Rhythmic patting, stroking

- Physical Security
  1. Swaddling
  2. Flexion with head support

- Auditory Stimulation
  1. Parent's voice
     a. Talking (high-pitched voice)
  2. Soft, rhythmic sounds
     a. Singing, humming, nursery rhymes
  3. Familiar sounds
     a. Sounds heard in utero
  4. Mechanical
     a. Music (distinct rhythms, 60–100 beats per minute)
     b. Intrauterine sounds
  5. White noise (monotonous sound that "drowns out" other sounds)

- Visual Stimulation
  1. Human face, with eye contact
  2. Mirrors, lights, ceiling fans, mobiles
  3. Pictures with black and white contrast
  4. Primary colors (especially red and yellow)

- Gustatory and Olfactory Stimulation
  1. Dripping colostrum or breastmilk on lips
  2. Offering clean finger to suck
  3. If parent not available, caregiver may wear parent's unwashed clothing

Source: Bocar, DL (1993). *Breastfeeding Educator Program,* p. 50. Reprinted with permission of Lactation Consultant Services, Oklahoma City, OK.

REFLEXES OF NEWBORNS

Infants are born with several reflexes that allow them to survive and that participate in cueing the infant for breastfeeding.

Rooting Reflex—Infants use the rooting reflex to locate the source of food. Touching or stroking the infants' cheeks causes them to turn toward the stimulus. This is a food-seeking response that allows them to find the breast. This response is evident by 32 weeks gestation (Amiel & Tison, 1967; Bu'Lock, Woolridge, & Baum, 1990). The infant should be placed with the lips in front of the nipple rather than in a position that requires turning toward the breast.

Suck–Swallow Reflex—The infant responds to touching on the lips by opening the mouth and sucking. Prenatally, infants have the ability to suck, as seen by ultrasound of infants sucking their thumbs. The suck reflex is evident by 24 weeks gestation (Herbst, 1981). Swallowing is seen in the fetus by 11 weeks (Miller, 1982) and sucking and swallowing is established by 32 weeks (Amiel & Tison, 1967; Bu'Lock, Woolridge, & Baum, 1990). By 37 weeks, the combination of sucking, swallowing, and breathing is well coordinated (Bu'Lock, Woolridge, & Baum, 1990).

Gag Reflex—Stimulation of the back two-thirds of the infant's tongue triggers a gag. This forceful movement of the tongue and reverse peristalsis of the pharynx brings forward anything that is dangerous to swallow. As the infant grows and develops, this reflex regresses to the back one-fourth of the tongue.

Transverse Tongue Reflex—The infant's transverse tongue reflex can be elicited by touch or taste stimulation applied to the side border of the tongue. The tongue will turn toward the stimulus. It is not a survival reflex, but it does help in the development of lateral tongue movements later on.

Palmomental Reflex—The palmomental reflex is a hand–mouth reflex. When the palm of the infant's hand is touched, the infant's chin wrinkles.

Babkins Reflex—Babkins reflex is another hand–mouth reflex. When the infant's palm is pressed, the mouth opens, the eyes close, and the head is brought forward.

Grasp Reflex—Infants are also born with a grasp reflex. The pressure of a finger placed against the finger flexors causes the baby to grasp the fingers and hold tightly. The grasp tightens when the baby sucks (Morris & Klein, 1987).

Assessing the Mother's Readiness to Breastfeed

PHYSICAL AND EMOTIONAL COMFORT

For many mothers, privacy during breastfeeding is a major issue. In assisting the mother, the lactation counselor should assess the mother's comfort with visitors, ask visitors to step out if indicated, place a sign on the door, turn off the telephone, etc., as needed for any individual mother. The physical and emotional comfort of the mother is very important. The mother should be advised to do the following prior to a feeding:

1. Empty her bladder.
2. Squeeze her buttocks together before sitting.
3. Sit on one side at a time to reduce episiotomy pain when sitting.
4. Take pain medication if indicated.
5. Have a warm, quiet room.

The mother and the health-care provider should wash their hands. The mother's nipples need no cleaning ritual because the Montgomery's tubercles secrete a bacteriostatic substance (sebum) to keep the nipples soft, pliable, and clean. The mother's normal flora is not harmful to the infant.

The health-care provider should assist the mother in getting into a comfortable position with her infant. Pillows and foot support are two maternal comfort measures. Pillows are useful in supporting the infant's weight and keeping the infant at breast level and in making the mother comfortable. They should be brought from home if the birthing facility provides only a limited number. Foot support, in the form of a stool, stack of books, the base of the tray table, etc., will elevate the mother's legs, improve her posture, and prevent back strain.

In conversing with the mother, the health-care provider should inspire confidence. She should avoid using phrases such as "Would you like to try to breastfeed?" Instead, the health-care provider should assure the mother that she will assist her and that the mother will learn the skills needed. Bocar (1993) lists common feelings that new parents experience and some suggestions for providing care (see Table 1B–2).

PSYCHOSOCIAL CONCERNS OF NEW PARENTS

New parents are overwhelmed with emotions over the birth of their infant. Many hours of thinking about the "big day" lead to expectations of a "dream experience," which may or may not be the case. In some areas of the country, births at home and at birthing centers have increased as parents try to exercise more control over the birth of their infant. The majority of births in developed countries still occur in hospitals, however. Parents are very sensitive to comments and nonverbal communication. Fatigue increases their vulnerability and feelings of inadequacy in the immediate postpartum period. First-time parents may be very rigid,

Table 1B–2   Common Feelings of and Care Suggestions for New Parents

COMMON FEELINGS

- Inadequacy, awkwardness, lowered self-confidence
- Vulnerability
- Sensitivity to comments/nonverbal communication
- Rigidity—"one BEST way to do things"
- Fatigue—feeling overwhelmed

SUGGESTIONS FOR PROVIDING CARE

- Provide *consistent* suggestions.
- Divide tasks into *easily mastered segments.*
- Provide *specific directions.* (Parents need concrete suggestions.)
- Offering many alternate choices may be overwhelming.
- Keep directions *simple.*
- Provide *specific, positive feedback.*
- Give lots of *praise.*
- *Personalize* infant—use given name frequently.
- Help place situation in *perspective.*
- Express *confidence* in their abilities.

Source: Bocar, DL (1993). *Breastfeeding Educator Program,* p. 59. Reprinted with permission of Lactation Consultant Services, Oklahoma City, OK.

perceiving one best way to handle baby-care activities. Books emphasizing parental control of infant care, such as *On Becoming BabyWise* by Ezzo and Bucknam (1995), have swept the country. Health-care providers may find the recommendations they provide regarding infant feeding are challenged by well-informed parents.

It is imperative that health-care providers understand the physiology of lactation to enable them to explain clearly to parents the "why" behind the "how to" in regard to breastfeeding. The importance of consistency in breastfeeding teaching in the early postpartum period cannot be overstated. Staff should not contradict one another. Directions to the parents should be kept simple, and tasks should be divided into easily mastered segments. Specific, positive feedback will boost the parents' self-confidence. Offering many alternative choices for positioning may be too confusing. Begin with one position; and after the mother has mastered it, teach another position.

The health-care provider must also respect the customs of other cultures. More and more, hospitals and clinics are caring for women who do not speak English or who follow practices different from those of mainstream American women. It is important to have access to translators and to provide written educational materials in a variety of languages.

PREFEEDING ACTIVITIES

Many new mothers feel pressured to "perform" at the first feeding, especially if overzealous or insensitive staff hover over the mother. It is appropriate for the caregiver to suggest relaxation techniques to calm an anxious or tired mother. Warm compresses to the breast or warm showers followed by breast massage may be helpful. The caregiver can provide full assistance to the mother or, if a family member or friend is available, the mother may be more comfortable with their assistance. See Table 1B–3 for ideas to elicit the milk-ejection reflex (MER).

Table 1B-3   Eliciting the Milk-Ejection Reflex

- Mother should be as comfortable as possible.
- Warm, quiet, private place. (Avoid interruptions.) Watch TV, read, and listen to soothing music (lullabies).
- Drink liquids (warm and noncaffeinated).
- Warm breasts.
  1. Warm and moist compresses × 5 minutes
  2. Warm showers
  3. Holding breasts over (or immersing breasts in) sink, basin, or bowl of warm water
- Massage breasts towards nipple.
  1. Fingertip (circular), diamond, and parallel massage
- Stroke and shake breasts.
- Look at baby (think of or look at pictures if separated).
- Use conscious relaxation, breathing techniques.
- Oxytocin
  1. Endogenous—nipple stroking and nipple rolling
  2. Exogenous—Syntocinon nasal spray (limited availability)
     a. Immediately before expressing

Source: Bocar, DL (1993). *Breastfeeding Educator Program*, p. 73. Reprinted with permission of Lactation Consultant Services, Oklahoma City, OK.

Support of the Breast

Hand positions can change the angle at which the nipple goes into the baby's mouth (see Figure 1B–1). The breast should not be handled in a manner that distorts it. The mother should support the breast as she presents it to the baby without altering where the breast normally falls at rest. Supporting and presenting the breast is a technique developed through practice. Knowing how to modify techniques to suit the mother's particular breast type can be the difference between success and poor results.

For women with large nipples, breast support will help the mother control the latch-on so that the baby is not allowed to latch-on until the mouth is open wide. Breast support may be necessary until the baby is older and able to nurse well without it. When this occurs varies but by the end of the first month most mothers find breast support unnecessary. Many mothers abandon this step too soon and develop sore nipples, so frequent reminding may be necessary in the hospital period.

C-HOLD

The C-hold (palmar grasp) position allows the mother to lift the breast and to guide her nipple into the infant's mouth (see Figure 1B–2). In the C-hold, the thumb is above the areola, and the remaining fingers are below and under the breast. Basic procedures for supporting the breast in the C-hold follow:

1. The breast is lightly supported with the hand, with four fingers underneath and behind the areola.
2. The thumb rests on top behind the areola. Gripping tightly or squeezing should be avoided.

Figure 1B–1

Hand positions

Source: Minchin, MK (1989). *Breastfeeding Matters—What We Need to Know About Infant Feeding*, p. 86. Victoria, Australia: Alma Publications. Reprinted with permission.

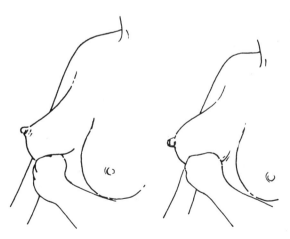

3. Supporting the breast in this manner:
   - Allows the mother to keep the nipple centered in the baby's mouth during latch-on.
   - Lifts the weight of the breast off the baby's chin.
   - Prevents the weight of the breast from dragging the breast out of the baby's mouth, causing nipple soreness.
4. The breast may need to be supported throughout the feed.
5. For women with large breasts, a rolled-up towel placed underneath the breast adds extra support and frees the mother's hand to help with latch-on.

SCISSORS HOLD

Normally the scissors hold is not recommended, but it can be used successfully by some women. The scissors or cigarette hold is a technique in which the nipple and areola are held between the index finger and middle finger. This method may prevent the baby from latching completely and may diminish drainage of the milk ducts.

NIPPLE SANDWICH

The nipple sandwich was developed by Barbara Heiser, a La Leche League leader, registered nurse, and board-certified lactation consultant. "The mother first uses

Figure 1B–2
Using the C-hold (palmar grasp) to latch-on infant
Source: Diane Davis, artist. Reprinted with permission.

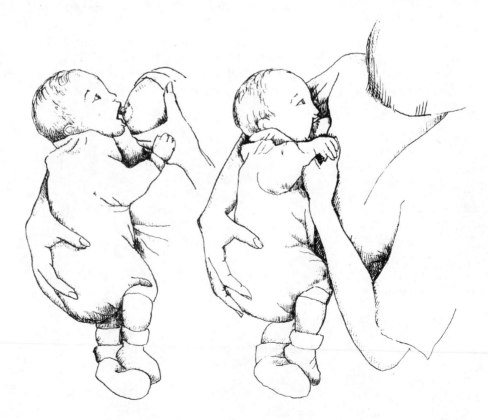

the C-hold to support the breast . . . then gently squeezes her fingers and thumb slightly together. This makes the areola oblong, instead of round. This means that there is now a narrower part for the baby to latch-on. The mother then pushes in toward her chest wall or rib. This helps the nipple protrude farther, which makes it easier for the baby to grasp. Finally, the mother pushes in with her thumb more than with her fingers. This makes the nipple point slightly upward toward the roof of the baby's mouth" (Mohrbacher & Stock, 1991). This type of support is beneficial for saggy, soft breasts or extremely large, firm breasts. It also may be useful for retracted or inverted nipples (see Figure 1B–3).

Figure 1B–3 Nipple sandwich

Source: Mohrbacher, N, Stock, J (1991). *The Breast-feeding Answer Book*, p. 53. Franklin Park, IL: La Leche League International. Re-printed with permission.

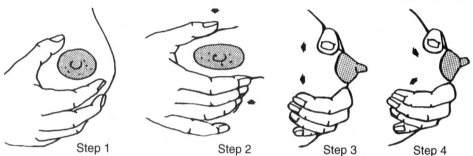

Step 1   Step 2   Step 3   Step 4

Step 1. Mother uses C-hold to support the breast. Both the fingers and the thumb should be behind the areola.

Step 2. Mother then gently squeezes her fingers and thumb together to make the areola area oblong, not round, giving the baby a narrower areola for latching.

Step 3. Mother then pushes in toward her chest wall, which causes the nipple to protrude farther.

Step 4. Mother pushes in with her thumb more than her fingers to make the nipple point slightly upward toward the roof of the baby's mouth.

Positioning

Breastfeeding can be done in a variety of different positions. Each is designed to bring comfort and efficiency to both the mother and the infant. Because the mother will spend many hours a day nursing her baby, she needs to know how to make herself comfortable in order to relax without straining her back, arms, neck, or legs. It's a good idea to suggest to the mother to designate a nesting area in her home where she will be comfortable and able to have privacy. It does not have to be in a bedroom. Many mothers prefer to establish themselves in the family room or den where they don't feel shut away from the activity and companionship of the rest of the family.

While the mother is in the hospital or clinic is an opportune time to experiment with various positions. Teach her how to manage these positions on her own, what to use to be comfortable, and how to tell others to help her. If you have an area for breastfeeding mothers in a clinic or office, be sure it is equipped with a table; a comfortable, stable chair; pillow support; and a stool.

CRADLE OR MADONNA HOLD

The cradle or madonna-hold position is the position commonly depicted in illustrations of women breastfeeding and is often the first position most women use. It is important for the LC to instruct the mother to

1. Sit as upright as possible, and to avoid slouching (see Figures 1B–4 and 1B–5).
2. Place supports (small pillows) at the lower back.
3. Place one or two pillows across the lap to lift baby to the level of the nipples.
4. Elevate the lap by placing the feet on a low footstool that is approximately 8 inches to 10 inches high. Many mothers find this eases lower back pain, takes pressure off the perineum, and helps in lifting the baby to the breast.
5. Uncover the breast to be used, exposing the breast well enough to place the fingers close to the ribs underneath to provide adequate support. Bras that restrict movement should be removed.
6. Place the baby on the pillows so that the head and body are level with the mother's nipple.
7. The baby's mouth faces the nipple, with the head resting on the mother's forearm. Forcing the head to rest on the crook of the mother's arm may strain the mother's shoulder.
8. Have the mother cradle the baby's bottom in her hand (depending on the length of the baby and the length of the mother's arm) with the baby's body facing the mother, tummy to chest. The baby's ear, shoulder, and hip will be in alignment. Babies should never breastfeed lying on their backs with their heads turned because this interferes with the alignment of the ear, shoulder, and hip.

Figure 1B–4

Nursing while sitting up

Source: Eiger, MS, Olds, SW (1987). *The Complete Book of Breastfeeding*, p. 125 (Wendy Way, artist). Copyright © 1987 by Marvin S. Eiger and Sally Wendkos Olds. Reprinted with permission of Workman Publishing Company, Inc., New York.

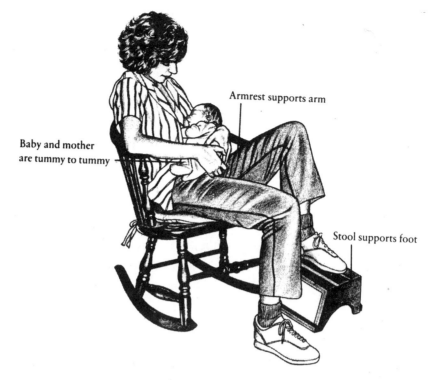

Figure 1B–5

Cradle or madonna hold

Source: Diane Davis, artist. Reprinted with permission.

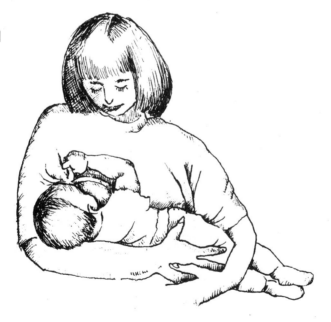

9. Hold the baby's body close, flexed across the mother's body. When babies are not held close in a curved position, they may hyperextend (flex backward), causing tonic neck fixation and very difficult latch-on. Note the body is flexed but the head should have room to extend slightly so the chin can be placed up under the lower part of the areola. This facilitates the infant's opening the mouth wide.

10. Now you're ready to begin initiating cueing and latch-on, which is discussed on pages 46–47.

MODIFIED CRADLE HOLD

The modified cradle hold is another position that is very helpful for mothers learning for the first time, for cases that require stabilization of the head, or for difficult latch-on (Figure 1B–6).

1. Proceed through steps 1–6 under the cradle position.
2. In step 7, the mother holds the base of the baby's head in her opposite hand (left breast/right hand). The body of the baby is aligned along the arm of the supporting hand. Fingers of the supporting hand should avoid touching the baby's cheek or face; this confuses the baby's rooting reflex.
3. The mother's opposite hand is now free to support the breast in the C-hold or nipple sandwich. This hold offers the mother better visibility and more control over baby's movements; and it facilitates easier latch-on.
4. Continue with steps 9 and 10 under the cradle position.

CLUTCH HOLD

Clutch hold (often called football hold—see Figure 1B–6) is good for women who

- Have large and/or pendulous breasts.
- Have flat, inverted nipples.
- Had a cesarean birth.
- Had a small or premature baby, or a baby that experiences difficulty latching on to the breast.
- Are nursing more than one infant at a time.
- Need to change positions because of sore nipples, mastitis, or clogged ducts.
- Desire stabilization of the infant's head.

Figure 1B–6
Modified cradle hold and clutch hold positions
Source: Diane Davis, artist. Reprinted with permission.

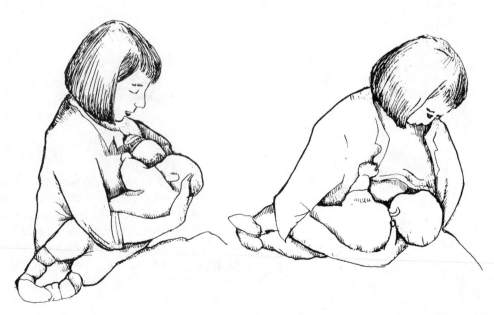

To position for the clutch hold:

1. Instruct the mother to sit upright in a firm chair or couch; support the back and legs as needed.
2. Place one or two pillows at your side to raise the baby to nipple height; avoid leaning down toward the baby.
3. Place the baby's bottom against the back of the chair or couch, with the back and neck along mother's forearm, supporting the baby's head in the mother's hand. If needed, use a rolled towel to wedge under mother's hand to prevent fatigue and the baby slipping off the breast. If the baby begins to push with his feet against the back support, place his bottom firmly against the support with his legs upright.
4. The mother holds the baby's body snuggled close to her side, with the mouth directly facing her nipple.
5. The baby's hands and arms can be tucked under large breasts, or the baby can be swaddled.
6. Now you are ready to initiate cueing and latching on as described on pages 46–47.
7. After latch-on, be sure the mother keeps the baby lifted to the breast throughout feedings and does not lean down onto the baby.

The clutch hold can be awkward for women with long limbs, slender bodies, and large babies or women with heavy breasts, short limbs, and small babies. Modification of this hold may be necessary for these mothers.

LYING-DOWN POSITION

Every mother should know how to breastfeed while lying down (see Figure 1B–7) before being discharged from the hospital or clinic. This position is good for

- getting more rest during night feeds.
- getting additional rest during the day.
- women who have had cesareans, epidurals, or difficult births.
- sore perineums.
- changing positions because of sore nipples, mastitis, or clogged ducts.

Figure 1B–7

Nursing while lying down

Source: Eiger, MS, Olds, SW (1987). *The Complete Book of Breastfeeding*, p. 125 (Wendy Way, artist). Copyright © 1987 by Marvin S. Eiger and Sally Wendkos Olds. Reprinted with permission of Workman Publishing Company, Inc., New York.

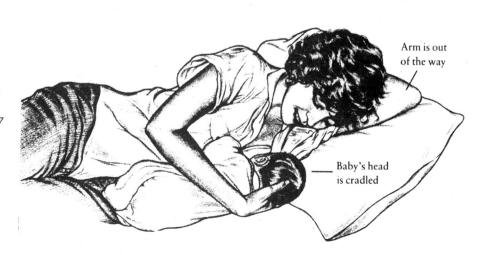

Many mothers have spent their entire breastfeeding experience sitting up for every feed because they were unaware that it was "OK" to breastfeed lying down. Most are grateful to be taught this sleep-saving technique.

1. Mother lies on her side, bolstered with pillows between her knees, at her lower back, and one or two under her head. For a sensitive abdomen, gently wedge a towel underneath for support.
2. The lower arm may be placed under the mother's head or she may use it to curve around the baby's back. The upper arm and hand are used to support the lower breast for latch-on.
3. Place the baby on his or her side, directly on the bed or couch facing the mother, mouth directly level with nipple. For women with large breasts, the baby's head can rest in the crook of the lower arm. Adjust for various mother–baby body combinations.
4. Place a rolled towel or pillow behind the baby's back to prevent rolling.
5. The baby's hips and legs are pulled close to mother's body.
6. Use the free upper hand to offer the breast and initiate latch-on.

It is helpful to know how to change breasts while remaining in a reclining position. To change breasts while lying down (see Figure 1B–8), remember the following:

Figure 1B–8

Transferring infant to the other breast following a cesarean birth

Source: Diane Davis, artist. Reprinted with permission.

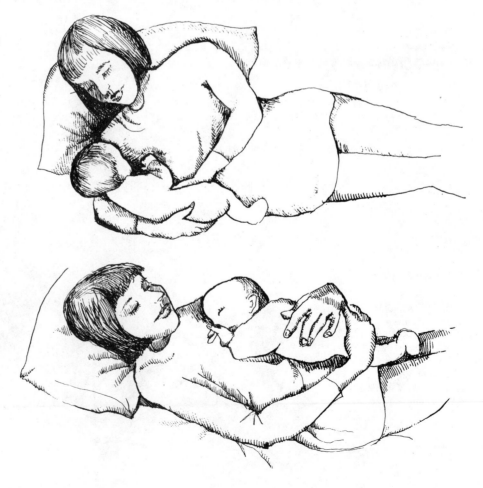

1. The caregiver can hold the baby while the mother turns over.
2. If the mother is able, she can hold the baby to her chest with one hand while she slowly turns over.
3. The mother stays on the same side and rolls forward slightly to offer the upper breast.

SPECIALTY POSITIONS

There are a number of specialty positions that can be used for gavage feeding; babies with neuromotor problems, cleft palate, or Down syndrome; babies who refuse one side, babies with weak muscle tone, and mothers with overactive milk-ejection reflexes. See Figures 1B–9 and 1B–10. Module 4, *The Management of Breast-feeding*, Chapter 3, provides more information on specialty positions.

Figure 1B–9

Positioning for over-active MER

Source: Diane Davis, artist. Reprinted with permission.

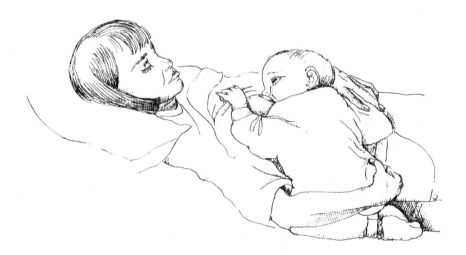

Figure 1B–10

Comfortable position for breastfeeding after a C-section

Source: Diane Davis, artist. Reprinted with permission.

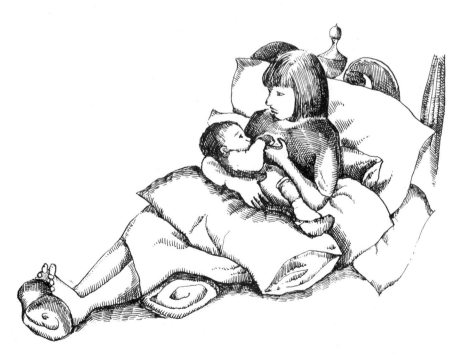

Cueing and Latch-on Techniques

Stroking the infant's cheeks or lips causes him or her to rotate the head toward the stimulus and open the mouth to search and suck. This is a rooting reflex. With correct positioning, the infant's mouth is placed in direct proximation to the nipple and areolar tissue. The infant responds to the touching on the lips by opening the mouth and sucking. This is the suck–swallow reflex.

Too much manipulation or touching about the infant's face is confusing and makes latch-on difficult. Grasping the baby by the head to turn him toward the nipple only causes him or her to turn in the direction of the pressure or hyperextend. Rather, when head support is necessary, do so by holding the base of the baby's head behind the ears. See Table 1B–4 for guidelines for cueing an infant for latch-on.

Reflexes may be suppressed or delayed by the use of pain medication or anesthesia during labor. Extended periods of mother/baby separation after birth may also cause diminished response (Widstrom et al., 1987).

Stimulating the rooting reflex is the first step in helping the baby to take the breast. Too often this step is done in a hurried manner, forcing the baby to fight and the mother to become frustrated. It is best to use the baby's natural trigger responses to initiate breastfeeding. When the mother learns to accomplish this step well, most of the common breastfeeding problems can be minimized. Many mothers benefit from physical assistance in addition to verbal instructions.

MANAGEMENT SUGGESTIONS

To assist the mother and baby with latch-on:

1. The helper needs to work at the same level with the mother, be relaxed and unhurried, and speak in reassuring tones.

Table 1B–4   Guidelines for Cueing Infant for Latch-on

- Mother lifts breast. Thumb is on upper aspect of breast, well behind areola. Index finger is on lower aspect of breast, well behind areola. Ideally, index finger is placed where her breast meets her chest wall, except when breasts are very large.
- Mother's fingers are placed on breast tissue, not areolar tissue. Areola is available for grasping by infant's mouth.
- Mother maneuvers her breast so that her nipple LIGHTLY touches her infant's lips. Tactile stimulus elicits the mouth-opening reflex.
- To accomplish a LIGHT touch, mother must allow space (approximately 1 cm) between infant's lips and her nipple tip. Pressing her baby's face very close to her breast prior to latch-on does not cue the mouth-opening reflex.
- When infant's mouth is opened WIDELY, mother lifts her entire breast from beneath and centers her nipple OVER her infant's tongue. Mother then pulls her infant close to accomplish latch-on in one motion.

Source: Bocar, DL (1993). *Breastfeeding Educator Program*, p. 150. Reprinted with permission of Lactation Consultant Services, Oklahoma City, OK.

Figure 1B–11

The rooting reflex

Source: King, FS (1992).
Helping Mothers to Breastfeed,
Revised Edition, p. 13. Nairobi, Kenya: AMREF. Reprinted
with permission.

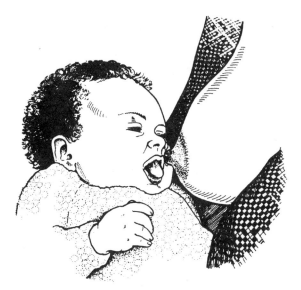

2. The mother tickles the baby's lower lip and waits for the baby to open his or her mouth wide and lift the chin. The mother may want to say "open" as she tickles the baby's lip. See Figure 1B–11 for an example of the rooting reflex. When the nipple touches near the baby's mouth, he or she opens his or her mouth and tries to find the nipple.

3. The baby is then quickly brought onto the breast in a swift movement.

4. When the nipple is placed deep into the baby's mouth and contacts the back of the hard palate, the baby will begin to suck. (Lubricating the nipple with expressed breastmilk may be helpful.)

5. The mother continues to support the breast, with her fingers at least two inches away from the areola, lifting the underside with four fingers.

6. Check that the baby's lips are flared out and tightly sealed against the breast, centered on the areola.

7. The baby's tongue should cup the breast and be visible just inside the lower lip. This can be checked by gently pressing a finger into the breast by the baby's lower lip and pulling the lip down.

8. The muscles above the baby's ears move rhythmically in response to the work of sucking.

9. Swallowing, interspersed with breathing, sounds like "cah-cah"; the baby's jaw moves with deep, piston-like strokes. After the baby initially latches on, he or she sucks rapidly to "call-up" the milk-ejection reflex in the mother. As the milk begins to flow, the baby's suck becomes rhythmic and slower than the "call-up" suck.

10. If the breast blocks the nose excessively (babies breathe through the flared sides of the nostril while at the breast), have the mother lift her breast and drop her shoulder or pull the baby's legs and body in closer to her instead of pressing down on the top of the breast (Mohrbacher & Stock, 1991).

Feeding Management

FEEDING DURATION

Each baby feeds at an individual rate based on temperament, physical well-being, and milk availability. Previous breastfeeding instructional material recommended limiting the duration of early feeds to two to five minutes per breast to avoid sore nipples. Current data, however, indicates that sore nipples are best prevented by correct positioning of the nipple in the baby's mouth. Because infants suck at their own rate, limiting feeding time decreases nutritional intake and interrupts the establishment of an adequate milk supply in the mother. Average feeding duration is 15 to 40 minutes total. The baby is allowed to feed on the first breast until the baby stops sucking, falls asleep, or needs to burp. Then the second side is offered, and the baby is allowed to nurse until satisfied. Feeding on only one breast per nursing session is not unusual and is an accepted practice.

Encourage the mother to study her baby's cues and to use her intuition during this training period. Every feed will not last the same amount of time; each will be determined by the degree of hunger and the sucking needs of the baby. Rigid adherence to a predetermined schedule impairs the natural cycle of supply and demand. Babies that are not allowed to nurse to satisfaction require supplementary feeds, and mother's milk supply decreases. Emphasize to the mother that she puts the baby on the breast, but the baby takes himself off.

BREASTFEEDING FREQUENCY

Previous material advised adherence to regularly spaced feeds every three to four hours. This advice was based on bottle-feeding routines. Because of the biological specificity and composition of human milk, frequent feeding patterns are recommended for human infants. Human milk is digested very quickly, and breastfed infants need to be fed more often than their counterparts fed manufactured milk. Average feeding patterns are every one and one half to three hours, allowing for appetite increases and growth spurts. As with feeding duration, the newborn's individual needs vary. Generally, 8 to 12 feedings during a 24-hour period are recommended.

REMOVING BABY FROM THE BREAST

When the baby does not come off the breast willingly, or the mother needs to switch breasts or rest, it is necessary to break the suction. Improper release damages the nipple tissue and cause sore nipples.

To release the suction, pull down on the baby's chin until the baby hears or feels release of the teat. The mother can use her index finger or pinky to wedge between the baby's gums. This will prevent the baby from slipping the nipple back in or chomping down to hold on.

The role of the health-care provider is to assist with feeding at the breast, including all of the following areas:

- Assess readiness
- Assist with positioning
- Assist with cueing and latching
- Assess the infant at the breast

This section provided information for the first three. The fourth area is covered in the next section of this module.

POST-TEST

For questions 1 to 4, choose the best answer.

1. Colostrum is available for the baby
    A. by the second day postpartum.
    B. at birth.
    C. two hours after birth.
    D. later in the mother who had a cesarean delivery than a vaginal delivery.

2. Skin-to-skin contact
    A. is not recommended immediately after birth.
    B. interferes with the motor development of the baby.
    C. is not recommended until after the infant has been removed for a physical exam and bath.
    D. is sufficient to maintain the healthy baby's body temperature.

3. The first feeding at the breast should occur as soon as possible because
    A. it will cause the infant to remain in a wakeful state for the next 12 hours.
    B. the sucking response is most intense during the first hour after birth.
    C. it keeps the mother from having uterine contractions.
    D. it puts the infant to sleep, so the physical exam by the physician can proceed more smoothly.

4. Crying can be described as
    A. the first indication of an infant's desire to feed.
    B. a harmless and naturally occurring process in newborns.
    C. a late hunger cue.
    D. having no effect on latch-on.

For questions 5 to 8, choose the best answer from the following key:
    A. Rooting reflex   C. Gag reflex
    B. Suck–swallow reflex   D. Babkins reflex

5. Reflex that helps the infant find the breast.

6. Reflex that can be stimulated by incorrectly performing a digital suck assessment.

7. Can be used to get the infant to open his mouth.

8. Is evident by 32 weeks gestational age.

For questions 9 to 12, choose the best answer.

9. Prior to a feeding, a new mother should
    A. not take pain medication.
    B. clean her nipple prior to offering the breast to the baby.
    C. give her infant a bottle of glucose water.
    D. empty her bladder, wash her hands, and find a comfortable position.

10. Eliciting the milk-ejection reflex is improved by
    A. cold compresses to breasts.
    B. drinking a beverage.
    C. using a nipple shield.
    D. massaging, stroking, and shaking the breasts.

11. This allows the mother to lift her breast and guide her nipple into the infant's mouth.
    A. Scissors hold
    B. Nipple shield
    C. C-hold
    D. Use of a rolled towel underneath the breast

12. These may prevent the baby from latching on completely and may diminish drainage of the milk ducts.
    A. C-hold and dimple ring
    B. Scissors hold and nipple shield
    C. C-hold and nipple shield
    D. Scissors hold and dimple ring

For questions 13 to 16, choose the best answer from the following key:

A. complete inversion of nipples	**C. difficult latch-on**
B. night feedings	**D. scissors hold**

13. Stabilization of head may help correct _____.

14. Lying-down position allows mother to rest during _____.

15. Choice of breast support can improve _____.

16. May block milk ducts from draining.

For questions 17 to 20, choose the best answer.

17. The duration of an individual feed
    A. should be a minimum of 30 minutes.
    B. will not vary over a 24-hour period.
    C. should be limited to prevent sore nipples.
    D. is determined by the baby's degree of hunger and sucking needs.

18. Breastfeeding frequency in the young infant
    A. can be increased by supplementing with manufactured milk.
    B. varies with individual babies.
    C. should be spaced every three to four hours.
    D. will be affected by maternal diet.

19. To cue the infant for latch-on, the mother
    A. presses the baby's face very close to her breast prior to latch-on.
    B. lightly tickles the infant's lower lip with her index finger.
    C. lightly tickles the infant's cheek with her breast.
    D. maneuvers her breast so that her nipple lightly touches her infant's lips.

20. All of the following may help with latch-on except:
    A. lubricating the nipple with expressed breastmilk.
    B. lightly touching the infant's lip with the breast.
    C. waiting until the infant is very hungry.
    D. repeating the word "open" while tickling the baby's lips.

SECTION C

Breastfeeding Assessment

Rebecca F. Black, MS, RD/LD, IBCLC
Donna Calhoun, BS, IBCLC

LEARNING OBJECTIVES

At the completion of this section, the learner will be able to do the following:

1. Assess the infant at breast for correct positioning, latch-on, sucking, and milk transfer.
2. State two anatomic characteristics specific to the infant that assist with breastfeeding.
3. Instruct the breastfeeding mother on how to assess audible swallowing while the infant is breastfeeding and explain the importance of this assessment.
4. Describe differences in expected stooling and urine patterns of the newborn and older infant.
5. List the steps to performing a digital suck assessment.
6. List three symptoms and signs in the infant that alert the clinician to intervene.
7. Describe two assessment tools that can be used to evaluate breastfeeding.
8. Describe two charting methods that can be useful in documenting encounters with breastfeeding women and their families.

OUTLINE

I. Feeding Physiology

A. Suckling and sucking

B. Nutritive and nonnutritive sucking

C. Sucking and swallowing by gestational age

  D. Full-term neonate coordination of sucking, swallowing, and breathing

  E. Infants' anatomic characteristics that are important to breastfeeding

  F. Stooling and urine patterns in infancy

  G. Appetite (growth) spurts

II. Functional Assessment of the Feeding

  A. Key factors in assessing breastfeeding adequacy

  B. Maternal and infant indicators of a good feed

  C. Assessing positioning, cueing, and latching

  D. Utilizing sucking patterns to assist breastfeeding assessment

  E. Suck assessment by digital exam

  F. When intervention is necessary

  G. Clinical indicators

  H. Assessment tools

  I. Documentation

PRE-TEST

For questions 1 to 4, choose the best answer.

1. Sucking is defined as the process whereby the infant stretches the breast tissue to form a teat that is pressed against the _____ with the _____.

    A. pharynx; tongue
    B. palate; tongue
    C. tongue; palate
    D. buccal fat pads; palate

2. The wavelike peristalsis of the infant's tongue during breastfeeding moves from

    A. front to back.
    B. back to front.
    C. left to right.
    D. right to left.

3. All of the following are true of nonnutritive sucking except:

    A. increases peristalsis.
    B. enhances digestive fluid secretions.
    C. occurs frequently during breastfeeding.
    D. should not be used to describe breastfeeding.

4. Sucking and swallowing are established by

    A. 36 weeks gestational age.
    B. 28 weeks gestational age.
    C. 32 weeks gestational age.
    D. 37 weeks gestational age.

For questions 5 to 9, choose the best answer from the following key:

A. Buccal fat pads   D. Appetite spurts
B. Stooling output   E. Weight
C. Urine output

5. _____ increases after colostrum changes into transitional milk due to increased milk volume.

6. _____ may not be evident in the premature infant.

7. _____ occurs frequently in a breastfed infant who is fed appropriately during the neonatal period.

8. _____ declines initially in most infants.

9. _____ can be accompanied by fussy behavior; frequent feedings resolve it.

For questions 10 to 13, choose the best answer from the following key:

A. Milk transfer   C. Audible swallowing
B. Areolar compression   D. Latch-on

10. _____ is the movement of milk from the mother's mammary glands to the infant's mouth.

11. _____ is the process that occurs when an infant opens the mouth widely with flanged lips and is brought to the breast.

12. _____ results from the rhythmic movement of the mandible so that a teat is formed.

13. _____ is not always evident in early feedings.

For questions 14 to 20, choose the best answer.

14. Maternal indicators of a good feed in the early postpartum period (first few days) include
    A. drowsiness, breast contractions, thirst.
    B. drowsiness, breast contractions, thirst, softening of the breast after a feeding.
    C. drowsiness, uterine contractions, thirst.
    D. drowsiness, uterine contractions, thirst, softening of the breast after a feeding.

15. Indicators of an adequate milk supply in a three-week-old infant include
    A. one to two bowel movements per 24 hours, swallowing for a sustained period during feeding, ½- to 1-oz. weight gain per week.
    B. three or more bowel movements per 24 hours, swallowing for a sustained period during feeding, ½- to 1-oz. weight gain per week.
    C. three or more bowel movements per 24 hours, swallowing for a sustained period during feeding, ½- to 1-oz. weight gain per day.
    D. one to two bowel movements per 24 hours, swallowing for a sustained period during feeding, ½- to 1-oz. weight gain per day.

16. Suck assessment by digital exam
    A. should be a part of each breastfeeding assessment.
    B. detects incorrect sucking action.
    C. requires the use of a syringe and feeding tube.
    D. is never recommended, for infection-control reasons.

17. The following conditions may decrease feeding frequency except:

    A. placid or lethargic baby.
    B. separation of mother and baby.
    C. use of nipple shield.
    D. supplementation with dextrose water.

18. Time restrictions at breast

    A. prevent sore nipples.
    B. have no effect on hyperbilirubinemia in the newborn.
    C. minimize milk leaking from breasts.
    D. decrease breast stimulation.

19. Lactation consultants can minimize their legal risk by all of the following except:

    A. obtaining consent for treatment.
    B. maintaining confidentiality.
    C. following through on service.
    D. pointing out hospital practices that interfere with breastfeeding to a patient.

20. Hollow cheeks and/or smacking sounds may signify

    A. an adequate areolar grasp and compression.
    B. an inadequate milk-ejection reflex in mother.
    C. that the tongue is drawn back behind the lower gum.
    D. an infant is experiencing feeding apnea.

Feeding Physiology

Feeding specialists have differentiated between suckling and sucking, which has led to confusion regarding the terminology used to describe breastfeeding. The terms suckling and sucking are defined separately, using function of the tongue and the age of the baby as criteria.

SUCKLING AND SUCKING

Suckling is the process whereby the infant stretches the breast tissue to form a teat, pressing the stretched areola against the palate with the tongue. Suckling is the earliest pattern observed in infants. The tongue moves backwards and forwards. This has been described as lick-sucking because of the extension–retraction of the tongue. Liquid or very soft food is drawn into the mouth by the rhythmic licking of the tongue and pronounced opening and closing of the jaw. Tongue protrusion does not extend beyond the lips and the most pronounced action is the backward phase of the movement (Morris & Klein, 1987).

Sucking is the second pattern to develop and begins at four to six months. The tongue moves up and down, the jaw makes a smaller movement, and the lips are firmly approximated (Figure 1C–1). Negative pressure builds in the mouth as a result of these coordinated movements. This has been described as pump-sucking (Morris & Klein, 1987).

Experienced breastfeeding clinicians do not agree with Morris and Klein that the infant's pattern of feeding at the breast changes over time (i.e., from suckling to sucking), but that the infant expands the ability to swallow a bolus of food without changing the way he or she feeds at the breast. Instead, the term *suckle* refers to what the mother does and the term *suck* refers to what the infant does at the breast. The mother suckles her infant with her breast. The infant sucks at the breast. Therefore, *sucking* will be used in this text to describe feeding at the breast by the infant. See Table 1C–1 for a description of the sucking action.

NUTRITIVE AND NONNUTRITIVE SUCKING

Another set of terms used to describe feeding is nutritive and nonnutritive sucking. These terms originated as operational definitions in psychology research for artificially fed infants (Wolff, 1968). *Nutritive* was defined as full and continuous milk flow and *nonnutritive* as alternating sucking bursts and rests during minimal milk intake.

Bowen-Jones, Thompson, and Drewett (1982) argue that these terms should not be used to describe breastfeeding, because one can never really know if milk is or isn't flowing. McBride and Danner (1987) proposed nonnutritive sucking to refer to spontaneous sucking without anything being introduced into the infant's mouth (which is common during sleep) or sucking prompted by a pacifier or finger being introduced into the infant's mouth without added liquid nutriment. Measel and

Figure 1C–1

Infant sucking at the breast

Source: Woolridge, MW (1986). The 'anatomy' of infant sucking. *Midwifery*, 2: 165. Reprinted with permission of Churchill Livingstone.

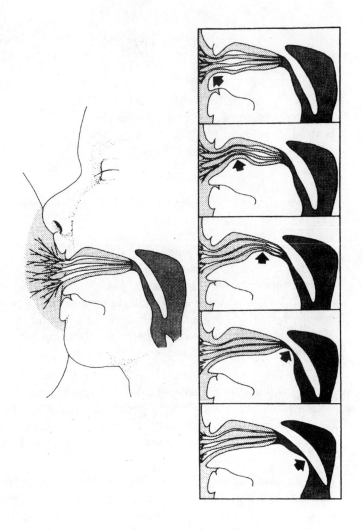

Table 1C–1 The Sucking Action

1. **Stretching the breast tissue to form a teat**

   A baby does not take just the nipple into his mouth. He takes a mouthful of the areola and the breast tissue beneath that contains the lactiferous sinuses. The baby must pull out or stretch the breast tissue into a "teat" that is much longer than the "resting" nipple. The nipple forms only one-third of this "teat." You can sometimes see the long, stretched breast tissue for a moment when the baby stops sucking.

2. **Pressing the stretched areola with the tongue against the palate**

   A wave (like peristalsis) goes along the tongue from the tip to the back near the baby's throat. The wave presses the milk out of the lactiferous sinuses into the baby's mouth so that he can swallow. You can often see the tip of the baby's tongue over the lower gum while he sucks. The tongue is "cupping" the breast. The buccal fat pads fill out the cheeks and meet the sides of the troughed tongue. This creates a negative pressure, which facilitates milk transfer. Suction helps to pull out the breast tissue and hold it in the baby's mouth. Suction does not remove the milk. It is the dynamics of a positive pressure–filled duct system attached to a negative pressure–filled oral cavity combined with the stripping of the teat by the tongue that removes the milk.

Anderson (1979) reported that nonnutritive sucking in premature infants increases peristalsis, enhances digestive fluid secretion, and decreases crying.

SUCKING AND SWALLOWING BY GESTATIONAL AGE

The fetus is reported to begin swallowing as early as 11 weeks gestation (Miller, 1982). The suck reflex is evident by 24 weeks (Herbst, 1981). By 32 weeks, the rooting response and linkage of sucking to swallowing is established (Amiel-Tison, 1967; Bu'lock, Woolridge, & Baum, 1990). By 37 weeks, the combination of sucking, swallowing, and breathing is well coordinated (Bu'lock, Woolridge, & Baum, 1990).

FULL-TERM NEONATE COORDINATION OF SUCKING, SWALLOWING, AND BREATHING

In utero, the infant has had two months to practice sucking and swallowing; so the first feeding at the breast is not its first experience with sucking and swallowing. What is new is the coordination of breathing with sucking and swallowing.

Ardran, Kemp, and Lind (1958) conducted the first studies in this area using radiographic means (before the dangers of such methods to the tissues were known). They contend that at the onset of the swallow, airflow is momentarily interrupted and then restored. Morris (1987) argues that the differences in the infant's oral anatomy enables respiration during swallowing. Several researchers used ultrasound to study the coordination of sucking, swallowing, and breathing in human infants between two and five days after birth (Bu'lock, Woolridge, & Baum, 1990; Weber, Woolridge, & Baum, 1986). Sucks occurred on their own or in combination with a swallow, but swallows did not occur on their own. None of the infants was observed to swallow while breathing. Younger breastfed infants (2–3 days old) swallowed intermittently, and breathing was independent of sucking and poorly coordinated with the swallows. Generally, swallowing caused an interruption in breathing with increasing age (4- to 5-day-old babies). Swallows were found in these ultrasound studies to occur consistently in the end-expiratory pause (between expiration and inspiration). Breathing responded to sucking rhythm and showed good coordination with swallowing.

The rate of milk flow is fast in the early stages of a breastfeed and gradually slows over the feed. Changes in the sucking rate at the breast with decreasing milk availability have been noted by clinicians. As suck–swallow units increase in response to milk flow, breathing becomes synchronized with sucking, so that the swallow occurs at the natural boundary between breathing out (expiration) and breathing in (inspiration).

Infant cyanosis is seen often in neonates, although the healthy neonate is reported to almost always recover spontaneously (Mathew & Bhatia, 1989). Infants are reported to be primarily nose-breathers (Morris, 1987), but they are capable of breathing through the mouth when necessary (Rodenstein, Perimutter, & Stanescu, 1985).

INFANTS' ANATOMIC CHARACTERISTICS THAT ARE IMPORTANT TO BREASTFEEDING

Mouth—The mouth is vertically short—when the infant's mouth is closed, the tongue touches the gums, buccal fat pads, and palate. The buccal fat pads (layers of fat in fibrous connective tissue) are located between the buccinator and masseter muscles. They provide stability and contribute toward the establishment of negative pressure in the infant's oral cavity during sucking.

Mandible—The infant's mandible (lower jaw) is receded and small. The infant's palate is short, wide, and slightly arched at birth. Rugae (corrugated transverse folds on the palate) and eminences of the pars villosa (tiny swellings on the oral mucosa of the lip's inner surface) facilitate holding the breast and areola in place (Ardran, Kemp, & Lind, 1958; Bosma & Showacre, 1975).

Pharynx—The infant's epiglottis is in closer proximity to the soft palate than is an adult's. It closes off the airway during swallowing. See Module 3, *The Science of Breastfeeding,* Chapter 1, for more information on the anatomy of the infant's oral cavity.

STOOLING AND URINE PATTERNS IN INFANCY

Stooling Output

In the breastfed infant, the stool changes from the black, tarry stools (meconium passage) of the first few days to the transitional stool, which begins lightening in color and becomes more liquid and less sticky. Breastmilk stool is very soft, liquid, or mushy and contains small curds at times. The color is greenish-yellow to mustard-yellow. The odor is described as "yeasty" and is less foul smelling than that of the infant fed manufactured milk.

The frequency of stooling increases after the first five to seven days. By one week of age, most exclusively breastfed babies will pass some stool during or immediately after nearly every breastfeeding. This pattern of frequent, scant bowel movements continues for four to six weeks (Weaver et al., 1988). Most clinicians believe a minimum of three stools per 24 hours should be expected in a well-nourished, breastfed infant in the first month of life. The frequency of stooling gradually declines, and the volume passed each time increases after the first month. Many infants stool an average of once every 4 to 12 days (Weaver, Ewing, & Taylor, 1988). When counseling parents concerned over the change in bowel habits, reassure them by reviewing the infant's well being. If the infant is gaining weight, appears contented, is in no discomfort or pain, and has a soft abdomen, there is usually no cause for alarm.

Lactobacillus bifidus found in human milk produces lactic acid from carbohydrates. Thus, the pH of the stool of the breastfed infant is low (5–6), and the acid environment discourages replication of enteropathogens like shigella, salmonella, and some E. coli. To families unfamiliar with breastmilk stools, the frequency and consistency may initially be confused with diarrhea. Diarrhea, however, is less prevalent in breastmilk-fed infants.

An inadequate stooling pattern may be the first symptom of weight gain problems or decreases in weight gain—patterns secondary to inadequate milk intake (Auerbach & Eggert, 1987). Organic conditions that affect stooling include Hirschsprung's disease and cystic fibrosis.

Urine Output

Infants are born with a surplus of extracellular fluid. In the colostrum stage of milk production, fluid intake via breastfeeding is small. Colostrum is measured in cubic centimeters, as opposed to ounces. The additional extracellular fluid present at birth can sustain the healthy term neonate until the increase in volume of the transitional milk. For these reasons, it is not uncommon for exclusively breastfed babies to have fewer wet diapers than their counterparts fed manufactured milk in the first few days of life.

Once the transitional milk arrives, urine output increases. Generally, infants have anywhere from 5 to 10 wet diapers per 24 hours. More frequent diaper changes are necessary if the mother uses cloth diapers than if she uses disposable ones. At a minimum, five to six wet disposable diapers per 24 hours and six to eight wet cloth diapers are expected. Urine volume decreases if the infant is taking in insufficient milk or has diarrhea and is losing excessive water in the stool. Concentrated urine is also more golden in color, and this color change should alert the mother to seek medical assistance.

Urine output alone, however, does not completely reveal the status of milk-intake adequacy. Infants can have problems with adequate weight gain and still produce wet diapers within the recommended range. This should alert the clinician to the need to check the style of breastfeeding used (i.e., mother breaks suction, moves infant to other breast prematurely) because the infant may be taking a large volume of foremilk from both breasts and thus not receiving the calorically dense hindmilk.

APPETITE (GROWTH) SPURTS

The symptoms of a growth spurt include a sudden increase in feeding frequency and duration and generalized fussiness in an infant who has previously been content after feedings and who has shown an acceptable pattern of weight gain. Mothers need to know when to expect appetite spurts: 7 to 10 days, three weeks, six weeks, three months, six months. The early appetite spurt at 7 to 10 days often coincides with the reduction of maternal breast swelling and may be misinterpreted by the mother as "losing my milk."

The management of appetite spurts includes frequent feeding and avoidance of supplementation. Until the recent work of Daly, Owens, and Hartman (1993), it was assumed that the milk-production rate took a period of days to change. Through computer-assisted imaging, they measured short-term milk-synthesis rates in a group of seven fully breastfeeding mothers. The authors concluded from their work that the mothers were capable of providing much more milk than their infants could consume. Further, they confirmed that the rate and volume of milk synthesis depended on the degree of breast emptying. Their results suggest that the breast can increase the rate of production as rapidly as the time between one interfeed interval and the next.

Well-meaning friends or relatives may question whether a baby is getting enough and may encourage a mother to supplement during a growth spurt. Anticipatory guidance can be helpful to mothers in alleviating their concerns of inadequate milk production. If they have already heard about when and what to expect with a growth spurt, they will be less likely to supplement with manufactured milk. When discussing growth spurts with mothers, remind them that they don't make more milk until they give some away. Thus, the quickest way to increase the milk supply (provided milk transfer is occurring) is to decrease the interfeed interval (i.e., nurse sooner and more frequently).

Functional Assessment of the Feeding

Assessment of breastfeeding involves good history taking, psychosocial evaluation, physical examination of the mother and infant, behavioral observation,
observation of breastfeedings, differential diagnosis, and the development of a
plan of care. This section covers information necessary for assessment, analysis,
and diagnosis of the breastfeeding relationship. Assessment tools to facilitate the
process are included. Treatment measures/interventions for specific problems are
outlined in Chapter 2 in this module; Module 3, *The Science of Breastfeeding*, Chapter 2; and Module 4, *The Management of Breastfeeding*, Chapters 1 through 3.

KEY FACTORS IN ASSESSING BREASTFEEDING ADEQUACY

The lactation consultant or caregiver can use four broad parameters to quickly
judge the adequacy of breastfeeding.

1. Is there evidence of milk transfer?
   - Swallowing is heard during feedings.
   - The frequency and duration of feeds are adequate.
   - The breast softens after a feed.
   - Breastmilk can be seen in and around the infant's mouth.

2. Is the mother comfortable?
   - The mother should not experience pain when breastfeeding.
   - No signs of pathologic engorgement exist.
   - The mother is relaxed and may also feel sleepy during feedings.

3. Is there sufficient infant output?
   - The infant has frequent bowel movement every 24 hours in the neona-
     tal period.
   - The infant has frequent wet diapers (5–6 for disposable diapers to 6–8
     or more for cloth diapers).

4. Is the infant gaining weight?
   - After the birth weight has been regained (usually by 10 days–2 weeks
     postpartum), the rate of weight gain is 4 to 7 ounces per week (½–1 oz.
     per day or 1–2 pounds per month).

The adequacy of the milk supply is not related to the length of time between feedings, the appearance of the milk (color, opaqueness, creaminess), or the frequency
of feedings. The frequency usually remains constant while exclusively breastfeeding (8–12 times in a 24-hour period) because infants are efficient feeders and sustain growth on approximately the same number of calories.

It is important to assess the adequacy of the mother's milk supply. Milk-supply
insufficiency is a common concern for mothers. Support for the concept of
autocrine control of milk production is strengthening as the importance of the
baby in regulating milk production becomes more evident (deCoopman, 1993).
Yet, the perception of insufficient-milk syndrome causes many mothers to quit

breastfeeding prematurely. Table 1C–2 lists indicators that can help assess the adequacy of the milk supply.

The position of the baby's head can also assist the breastfeeding assessment. While we often flex the baby's body through swaddling, we must be careful to allow the range of motion needed for the head of the infant to be correctly positioned. (See Figure 1C–1.) Some lactation consultants believe the head of the infant extends back slightly with the chin leading the open mouth to latch-on to the breast (Minchin, 1989b). Others argue the head is neither extended or flexed but is in a neutral position (Chele Marmet, personal communication, 1996).

Visual inspection of the breast during feeding can be helpful. The areolar tissue flattens and elongates to fill the oral cavity of the baby. See Figure 1C–2 for a visual depiction of how the shape of the breast changes during a feeding.

MATERNAL AND INFANT INDICATORS OF A GOOD FEED

The lactation consultant, nurse, nutritionist, or peer counselor can determine how a feeding is going by observing and listening to the mother and the infant. The mother may comment on uterine contractions in the early days of breastfeeding as oxytocin is released by her pituitary gland in response to the infant's suck. The infant's gums compress the fourth intercostal nerve in the mother's breast, which signals the pituitary to release oxytocin. Multiparas often report more intense uterine contractions. The breastfeeding counselor can reassure the new mother of the positive benefits of the uterine contractions and instruct her to expect the discomfort to lessen gradually over a few days.

Drowsiness during a feeding is another side effect reported by mothers. Hormone release contributes to the relaxation experienced by the mother during a feeding. It may be especially helpful in the early days after delivery to encourage the

Table 1C–2   Indicators of Adequate Milk Supply

Swallowing heard

Feedings are comfortable

Nursing 8 or more times each 24 hours (every 2–3 hours)

Infant swallows for at least 10 minutes

Breasts less full after nursing (after engorgement resolves)

Infant ends the feedings

Infant indicates satiety after feeding
- Infant "falls" away from breast in relaxed state
- Mother does not end feedings (no clock watching)

Infant displays contentment between MOST feedings

Frequent bowel movements
- At least 3 each 24 hours for first month
- 6 or more wet diapers each 24 hours
- Nonconcentrated urine (with no water or juice supplements)

Infant gains 4 to 7 ounces each week (½–1 oz./day)

Source: Bocar, DL (1993). *Breastfeeding Educator Program,* p. 78. Reprinted with permission of Lactation Consultant Services, Oklahoma City, OK.

Figure 1C–2

The changing curve of the postpartum breast during feeding

Source: Minchin, MK (1989). *Breastfeeding Matters—What We Need to Know About Infant Feeding*, p. 94. Victoria, Australia: Alma Publications. Reprinted with permission.

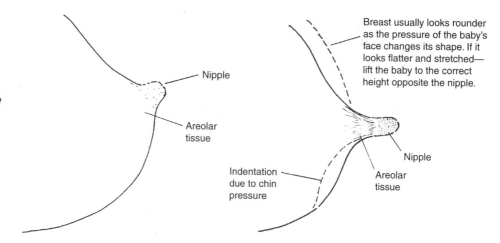

Nipple

Areolar tissue

Breast usually looks rounder as the pressure of the baby's face changes its shape. If it looks flatter and stretched— lift the baby to the correct height opposite the nipple.

Indentation due to chin pressure

Nipple

Areolar tissue

mother to breastfeed while in a reclining position. In a comfortable reclining position, the mother can allow the drowsiness she experiences to relax and quiet her emotionally as well as physically.

Thirst functions in response to hormones that are regulated by the kidney. When the antidiuretic hormone is released into the blood, the body conserves water; and thirst is "turned on." The production of human milk in the alveolar cell uses water, which in effect increases the antidiuretic hormone and thus increases thirst. Breastfeeding mothers notice that they are feeling thirsty and can generally maintain their fluid needs by responding to their own thirst.

A visual cue of milk transfer and a good feed is the softening of the breast after a feeding. In the immediate period after delivering, when the mother is producing colostrum, the breast is always soft. Colostrum is available in very small amounts, and there is minimal swelling of the breast in this stage of lacation. The breast will usually experience slight fullness as lactose is secreted into the milk and transitional milk is being produced. Lactose pulls more water into the breastmilk, and the volume of milk increases. Therefore, the softening of the breast after a feed is visually useful as a determinant of a good feed only after the colostrum period.

Infant indicators of a good feed include obvious output measurements such as regular stool and urine output. Most clinicians agree that stooling is most helpful in the first few days to determine whether the infant has received colostrum because urine output will be scant until the milk volume increases, as we've discussed.

The swallowing of milk by the infant at the breast is audible once the milk volume has been established. The swallowing sound is often described as "cah, cah." When there are questions about milk transfer, the breastfeeding counselor can kneel by the mother and infant pair with her ear close to the breast. It is helpful if the feeding environment is quiet—turn off radios, televisions, etc., that may impair the counselor's ability to hear the infant swallowing. Swallowing is heard between the expiration and inhalation phases of breathing. There may be several sucks before a swallow, depending on the flow rate of the milk. A section on utilizing sucking and swallowing patterns to assist breastfeeding assessment appears later in this chapter.

Flexion of the arms by the infant's side places the hand in close proximity to the mouth. It also alerts the clinician to a hungry baby. One positive physical sign of a good feed that an infant provides is the relaxation of the infant's arms during a feed. When combined with an infant who releases the breast spontaneously, the counselor can assume the infant is satisfied. How long the infant remains satiated varies from infant to infant and even varies within an individual infant.

Finally, weight gain is an outcome measure that confirms the adequacy of feedings over time. The expected pattern of weight gain varies depending on the age of the baby. In the neonatal period, most clinicians expect a breastfed infant to regain the birth weight by two weeks and like to see a ½- to 1-ounce daily gain in early infancy. Expected gains in weight, length, and head circumference are discussed in Module 4, *The Management of Breastfeeding*, Chapter 1.

Table 1C–3 summarizes the maternal and infant indicators of a good feed.

ASSESSING POSITIONING, CUEING, AND LATCHING

In the previous section of this chapter on feeding at the breast, the steps to position, cue, and latch an infant to the breast were described. The counselor assessing the feeding must rely on the visual sense to identify potential problems with positioning and cueing and on the auditory sense to assess latching. The mother who is in a sitting position needs to be made comfortable by supporting her arms and back. Depending on the height of the chair seat, the mother may need foot support as well. It is important to maintain the natural curvature of her spine to prevent muscle spasms in the back that may result from extended feeding without arm, back, and/or feet support. The presence or absence of arms on a chair or the weight of the arms may determine whether a pillow is needed to support the weight of the infant being held for feeding. Feeding holds that place the arm, wrist, or shoulder in an unnatural position should be avoided and corrected by the counselor during feeding assessment. The mother's body posture is an important indicator of good positioning. Leaning over the baby or the elevation of one or both shoulders during a feeding reveals problems with positioning. The following are signs that a baby is sucking in a good position (King, 1992):

- The baby's whole body is facing his mother and is close to her.
- The baby's face is close up to the breast.
- The baby's chin is touching the breast.
- The baby's mouth is wide open.
- The baby's lower lip is curled outward.

Table 1C–3 Indicators of a Good Feed

Maternal	Infant
• Drowsiness • Increased uterine contractions (in the immediate postpartum period) • Thirst • Softening of the breast after a feeding (after physiologic engorgement has subsided)	• Swallowing • Relaxed body—arms by side • Satisfied after feed • Frequent urine output • Regular stooling • Adequate weight gain

- There is more areola showing above the baby's upper lip and less areola showing below the lower lip.
- You can see the baby taking slow, deep sucks.
- The baby is relaxed and happy and is satisfied at the end of the feed.
- The mother does not feel nipple pain.
- You hear the baby swallowing.

The following are signs that a baby is sucking in a poor position (King, 1992):

- The baby's body may be turned away from his mother's.
- The baby's chin is separated from the breast.
- The baby's mouth looks closed.
- The baby's lip points forward.
- You see too much areola, including below the lower lip.
- The baby takes many quick, small sucks.
- The baby may fuss or refuse to feed because he or she is not getting enough breastmilk.
- The mother may feel nipple pain.
- The baby's mouth may make a smacking sound as he or she sucks.
- The nipple may look flattened at the end of a feed and it may have a line across the tip.

Maher (1988)* listed these indicators of effective positioning, cueing, and latching:

1. The mother is comfortable with her arms and back supported.
2. The mother does not lean over the baby.
3. When using the cradle hold, the baby is chest to chest, the knees are to the mother's other breast.
4. The baby's stomach is pulled in close to the mother.
5. The baby's ear, shoulder, and hip are in a straight line.
6. The mother holds her breast comfortably with relaxed shoulders and fingers positioned so that there is room around the areola for the infant's chin.
7. The baby responds to the tickle of her breast on his lower lip by opening the mouth wide.
8. The mother experiences the tugging of the suck, and may notice tingling or a "pins and needles" sensation indicative of a milk ejection reflex (see Figure 1C–3).
9. Audible swallowing is noted.

Table 1C–4 lists various ways to assess latch-on. Figure 1C–4 shows

A. a baby sucking in a good position.
B. a good sucking position. The breast is stretched into a "teat" in the baby's mouth.
C. the wave going along the tongue to press the milk from the lactiferous sinuses.

*Source: Maher, SM (1988). *An Overview of Solutions to Breastfeeding and Sucking Problems*. La Leche League International: Franklin Park, IL, pp. 5–6. Reprinted with permission.

Figure 1C–3

Baby bottle-sucking the breast (*left*) and baby actively sucking the breast (*right*)

Source: Minchin, MK (1989). *Breastfeeding Matters—What We Need to Know About Infant Feeding,* p. 92. Victoria, Australia: Alma Publications. Reprinted with permission.

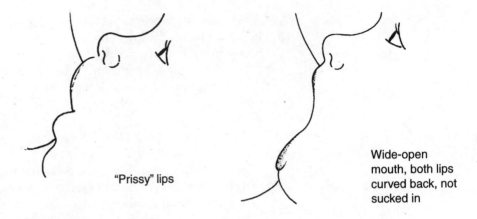

"Prissy" lips

Wide-open mouth, both lips curved back, not sucked in

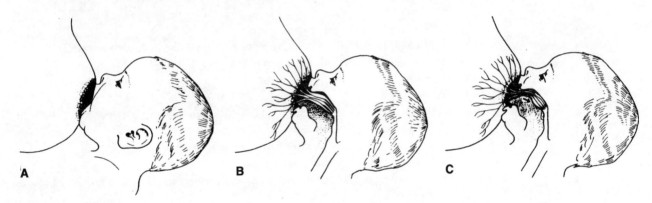

Figure 1C–4   How the baby sucks—good positioning
Source: King, FS (1992). *Helping Mothers to Breastfeed,* Revised Edition, p. 14. Nairobi, Kenya: AMREF. Reprinted with permission.

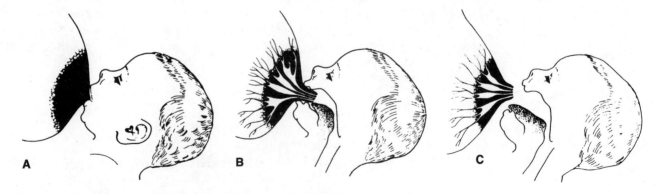

Figure 1C–5   How the baby sucks—poor positioning
Source: King, FS (1992). *Helping Mothers to Breastfeed,* Revised Edition, p. 15. Nairobi, Kenya: AMREF. Reprinted with permission.

Table 1C–4   Assessing Adequacy of Latch-on

Infant's mouth should be opened widely (2.0–3.0 cm).
  • Facilitate wide mouth opening
  • Maintain breast support throughout the feeding (through approximately 42 weeks gestational age).
  • Keep infant's nose and chin touching breast.

Infant's lips should be flanged outward.
  • Infant relaxes after sucking begins and milk is obtained.
  • As infant's body relaxes, mouth relaxes and opens more widely; lips become more flanged. If lips remain turned inward, nurse or mother can manually turn lips outward to increase maternal and infant comfort.

Mouth seal should be adequate to create sufficient intra-oral negative pressure (suction) to retain nipple within infant's mouth and to facilitate refilling of lactiferous sinuses.
  • No gap at the corner of the infant's mouth should be noted.

Infant's tongue should be troughed (curved) beneath areolar tissue and extended beyond the lower gumline.

Areolar tissue should be drawn into the infant's mouth as evidenced by less areolar tissue being visible after latch-on than prior to latch-on.
  • The nipple and areolar junction should not be visible.

Source: Bocar, DL (1993). *Breastfeeding Educator Program*, p. 65. Reprinted with permission of Lactation Consultant Services, Oklahoma City, OK.

Figure 1C–5 shows

  A. a baby sucking in a poor position.
  B. a poor sucking position. The baby is sucking only the nipple and the tongue is held back in the mouth.
  C. a baby opening his mouth to take the breast. The nipple is aiming at his palate. His lower lip is aiming well below the nipple.

UTILIZING SUCKING PATTERNS TO ASSIST BREASTFEEDING ASSESSMENT

The preconditions for successful breastfeeding include intact and functioning maternal breast(s) and infant oral cavity anatomy, and no metabolic disease or other condition in the mother that affects milk production or milk intake. It is of the highest biological priority for the infant to obtain milk and to stimulate future milk production.

Sucking patterns can provide information on how the feeding is going. Sucking at the breast can be characterized by the quality of the suck. Between 1960 and 1970, developmental psychologists looked at sucking patterns as clues to development. The majority of this research, however, was done on artificial teats. The researchers found it very difficult to switch off babies' desire to suck even with a distasteful source. When an infant is given a choice, the infant will express a choice for the better tasting one (higher sucrose). This is interesting because lactose has almost no variability once milk is established. Colostrum is lactose-free. No data is available on whether the coming in of transitional milk, the subsequent increase in volume, the new presence of lactose, and the duration of the infant's sucking at this time are interrelated.

Does Milk Flow Influence the Sucking Rate?

Woolridge (1986) has looked at what he defines as the burst/pause relationship to provide information on how sucking rates change in response to milk-flow changes. *Bursts* are periods of sucking that may or may not be associated with a swallow. *Pauses* are gaps between bursts of sucking.

Infants suck and swallow based on milk flow with a frequency of about one per second when breastmilk is actively flowing. If the milk-flow rate slows or stops, the rate increases to about two per second (Wolff, 1968). The sucking rhythm is well coordinated with swallowing so that 1:1:1 sequence of coordinated cycles of sucking, swallowing, and breathing occur (Bu'Lock, Woolridge, & Baum, 1990; Weber, Woolridge, & Baum, 1986; Wolff, 1968). When an increase in milk flow occurs, the infant decreases the rate of sucking. Fluctuations can be observed during different stages of feeding by observing changes in the infant's burst–pause patterns.

At the start of the feed, there is an inverse relationship between burst length and pause length—long bursts of sucking and short pauses. At low-flow rates, short bursts of sucking that tend to be disjointed and uninterrupted by pauses are observed. Toward the end of the feeding session, the relationship is positive—with long bursts followed by long pauses.

These investigations by developmental physiologists have led to many questions for which there are as yet no answers:

- Is the flow regulating the sucking pattern or is the nature of the suck regulating the flow?
- Does sucking intensity relate to milk removal?
- How do milk fat content and infant satiety change the burst–pause patterns of sucking?
- How do sucking patterns relate to hormonal release?
- To what extent can the mother disrupt the milk flow by distorting the breast (with an electric pump or by hand positioning)?

The breast is a three-dimensional structure and not all the ducts drain at the same rate or start emptying at the same time. Putting the baby to where the breast is naturally, to avoid manipulating the breast in a way that disrupts the flow of milk, is an important tip for mothers. If a baby at the breast exhibits a very fast pace of sucking interrupted by very frequent pauses, the feeding is not going well. Often providing the breast with support, where none was given before, or adjusting positioning, can bring about an immediate change in the sucking pattern of the baby.

SUCK ASSESSMENT BY DIGITAL EXAM

Sucking problems can arise from four basic problem areas:

1. *Innate*—thumb sucking in utero; illness
2. *Prematurity*—neuromotor–neuroendocrine dysfunction
3. *Genetic*—short frenum–frenulum; other anatomical variation in infant's oral cavity or mother's breast
4. *Iatrogenic*—early introduction of artificial teats, causing nipple confusion; intubation of premature infants

When problems with sucking are evident by visual evaluation of several feedings, a digital examination of the infant's oral cavity may be appropriate. It is warranted in cases of difficult latch-on or sucking dysfunction, as assessed by a clinician experienced in the technique of digital examination of the infant's oral cavity. The procedure is to position the infant with the head and shoulders slightly elevated (to mimic the feeding position) and, with a nonlatex gloved index finger (nail side down), tickle the infant's lower lip. This will elicit the mouth-opening reflex. Gently touch the tip of the tongue and note troughing or cupping of the tongue around the finger. Allow the infant to "pull" the finger into the mouth. To elicit a suck, apply slight downward pressure on the posterior tongue and stroke rhythmically to stimulate the suck (Bocar, 1993). Gently applied pressure to the junction of the hard and soft palate may elicit a suck (Marmet & Shell, 1984). Occasionally, enticement with water in a syringe or feeding tube may be necessary to elicit the sucking response. See Table 1C–5 for indicators of correct and incorrect sucking during a digital suck assessment.

Module 4, *The Management of Breastfeeding*, Chapter 3, discusses retraining and correcting a dysfunctional suck. Also, Riordan and Auerbach (1993), Marmet and Shell (1984), McBride and Danner (1987), Ross (1987), and Bocar (1993) all describe how to retrain a dysfunctional suck: Consult these references before performing a digital suck assessment and implementing suck training.

WHEN INTERVENTION IS NECESSARY

When breastfeeding does not proceed smoothly, it is necessary to distinguish between normal breastfeeding activity and abnormal activity in order to know when further help is needed. In the past, many mothers were not given help and weaned abruptly from the breast to the bottle. Now that much research and exper-

Table 1C–5   Digital Suck Assessment

Correct Sucking Action	Incorrect Sucking Action
• Tongue is beneath examining finger. • Tongue extends over mandibular alveolar ridge (lower gumline), and tongue curls around finger. • Complete seal is formed around examining finger. • Noticeable negative pressure is exerted on finger. • Rhythmic pattern of suck is noted, with anterior to posterior peristaltic motion.	• Tongue is against hard palate (on top of examining finger). • Tongue "rakes" across (pushes against) examining finger. • Tongue may push finger out of mouth (tongue thrust). • Back of tongue is elevated. Gagging may occur. • Tongue does not extend over lower gumline; infant "bites" with gums. • No organized, rhythmic motion is noted. • Complete seal is not formed around finger. • Weak or no suction occurs.

Source: Bocar, DL (1993). *Breastfeeding Educator Program*, p. 67. Reprinted with permission of Lactation Consultant Services, Oklahoma City, OK.

tise has improved breastfeeding knowledge, other measures are available to avoid weaning and to maintain the nursing relationship.

Infant-related problems with the breastfeeding process include refusal of the breast, sucking difficulties and/or dysfunction, nipple confusion, weak suck, ankyloglossia, tongue thrusting, tongue retraction, tonic bite reflex, and latch-on difficulties. Problems that mothers sometimes encounter related to the breastfeeding process include engorgement, plugged ducts, sore nipples, inadequate milk supply, and mastitis. Maternal information, attitude, motivation, feelings, health, and support and infant health and behavior in turn influence the above factors (Ellis, Livingstone, & Hewat, 1993).

CLINICAL INDICATORS

Intervention by a skilled practitioner is necessary for latching, cueing, and positioning difficulties; suck dysfunction; and failure to thrive secondary to insufficient milk. The following are symptoms of these problems:

- Fretful, uncontented after feeding
- Refusing one side
- Pulling away
- Mouth closes upon latch-on
- Won't latch-on
- No audible swallowing
- Dimpling in cheeks while sucking
- Poor suction/losing suction
- Biting
- Difficulty restarting
- Clicking while sucking
- Tongue not visible over lower gum
- Pursed lips
- Continuous flutter sucking
- Flexion of arms throughout feeding
- Feedings last more than one hour (nursing time, not nursing and sleeping time)
- Infant wants to nurse every hour (pattern last longer than 24–48 hours)
- Less than three bowel movements per 24 hours in first week
- Less than six to eight wet cloth diapers or five to six disposable diapers (per 24 hours)
- Loss of more than 10% of birth weight
- Failure to regain birth weight by 10 days to two weeks
- Intensified nipple soreness; sudden appearance of nipple soreness
- Pathologic engorgement in the mother

Table 1C–6 summarizes clinical situations that may increase the need for intervention from a skilled caregiver.

Table 1C–6   Clinical Indicators and How They Impact Breastfeeding

Clinical Indicators	Impact on Breastfeeding
Maternal infection, trauma, hemorrhage, illness, medications	May delay baby going to breast; systemic trauma may delay lactogenesis
Forceps, vacuum extraction, cesarean section, asphyxia, anesthesia, medications, caput succedaneum	Babies have been clinically observed to breastfeed poorly.
Weight in relation to gestational age of baby	Small for gestational age (SGA) babies (underweight, full term) may show poor muscle tone, poor sucking and rooting and stress when handled.
Large amounts of intravenous fluid with high concentrations of dextrose given during labor	Fluid may shift from mother to baby (Keepler, 1988) and cloud the calculation of birth weight and weight loss.
Delay in initiating lactation	Reduces stimulation to breast. Places infant at risk for feeding difficulties if nipple-fed during delay. May contribute to pathological engorgement if expressing of milk by mother not begun.
Separation of mother and baby	All items as stated for delay in initiating lactation. Mother does not learn to read hunger cues. May affect bonding.
Jaundice, phototherapy, supplemental fluids	Baby may feed lethargically. Water temporarily suppresses appetite, causing lengthening of feeding interval, leading to increased bilirubin levels (Auerbach & Gartner, 1987).
Use of nipple shields	Reduces stimulation to the nipple and areola, which decreases the milk supply (Amatayakul et al., 1987; Auerbach, 1990; Jackson et al., 1987)
Retained placental fragments, inadequate feeding frequency, improper sucking stimulus to breasts	Late onset of milk production (change from colostrum to higher-volume transitional milk delayed)
Pathological engorgement	Normal or physiological engorgement is necessary for lactogenesis. Pathological engorgement can lead to pressure atrophy of alveoli and permanent reduction in milk-making capacity of the breast (Lawrence, 1989).
Environmental stress can inhibit afferent arm of pathway that elicits milk-ejection reflex.	Loss of maternal reflexes of milk dripping, areolar fullness, tingling or full sensations of breasts
Milk inspissation (increased thickness or decreased fluidity secondary to fluid absorption), i.e., it remains in breasts (Weichert, 1980)	Cramping or shooting pains in breasts after feedings, breast fullness or ropy texture after feedings
Long intervals between feedings; few feedings per 24 hours	Intervals of greater than 2 to 3 hours or less than 6 to 8 total feedings per 24 hours can interfere with prolactin cycling, leading to engorgement, nipple problems, and less milk removal from breast.
Time restrictions at breast	Contributes to jaundice in newborn and use of supplements, does not prevent sore nipples, decreases breast stimulation and can lead to slow weight gain in baby
Scheduled feedings	Mother may miss infant behavioral feeding cues (Ellis, 1986; Hales, 1981); can lead to poor feeding if baby is awakened from a deep sleep.
Poor positioning of baby at breast, with trunk or neck hyperextended; sensory or orally defensive baby; long intervals between feedings; flat nipples; engorged areola with difficult latch-on; neurologic immaturity; neurologic damage (McBride & Danner, 1987)	Infant behavior at breast described as frantic, resists breast, irritable, pulls away or arches off, stops and starts, difficult latch-on, falls asleep after a few sucks.
Sucking dysfunction or disorganization (smacking or clicking when feeding, loses suction and slides off breast)	Baby may feed frequently to make up for small amounts received at each feeding.

continued

Table 1C–6 Clinical Indicators and How They Impact Breastfeeding *continued*

Clinical Indicators	Impact on Breastfeeding
"Good," placid baby that sleeps through night, has long daytime stretches of sleep (four or more hours between feedings), does not cry to be fed frequently	Baby may be underfed and calorie-deprived, leading to increased amount of sleeping and lethargic nursing. Baby may not give clear feeding cues to parents.
Supplementation with water, dextrose water, formula, juice	Supplements can decrease milk supply, prolong feeding intervals, and confuse sucking patterns.
Maternal responsibilities	May contribute to fatigue and decreased milk supply
Physical characteristics of infant, such as clefting, facial nerve paralysis, short frenulum, high or grooved palate	May make latch-on difficult
Poor muscle tone	May contribute to ineffective sucking and disinterest in feeding
Eczema accompanied by poor feeding and fussiness	May mean intolerance or allergy to cow's milk in maternal diet
Hollow cheeks, smacking sounds, small or large jaw excursions	May indicate tongue is drawn back behind lower gum and/or tongue and jaw not working as a unit
Babies with cardiac problems, SGA, or preterm infants, especially those with bronchopulmonary dysplasia	May have breathing irregularities, feeding apnea, circum-oral cyanosis

Source: Walker, M (1989). Functional assessment of infant breastfeeding patterns. *Birth,* 16(3):140–46. Reprinted by permission of Blackwell Scientific, Inc.

ASSESSMENT TOOLS

The care of nursing mothers and infants requires a unique form of interaction from the health-care professional. Even though it may be necessary to assess and direct the process, the practitioner must be careful not to diminish the participation of the mother. Awkwardness may inhibit the mother's ability to interact comfortably with her baby, and she will benefit from many encouraging comments.

Breastfeeding requires practice to become an instinctive routine. Consequently, assisting the mother to get off to a good start will help each feed to be pleasurable. During the early period when the mother is learning to breastfeed, the practitioner needs to observe a complete feed in order to detect any problems. Assessments should not be done during the first feed following birth, when mother and baby are getting acquainted. Too much interference at this point will diminish the mother's confidence and innate knowledge.

Several assessment tools for feeding evaluation have been published, including the Systematic Assessment of the Infant at the Breast (Shrago & Bocar, 1990), the Mother–Baby Assessment (Mulford, 1992), the Vancouver Breastfeeding Centre Tool (Ellis, Livingstone, & Hewat, 1993), the Infant Breastfeeding Assessment Tool (Matthews, 1988), the B-R-E-A-S-T Observation Form (Armstrong, 1990), and the LATCH Tool (Jensen, Wallace, & Kelsay, 1994). Reliability testing of these breastfeeding tools is underway, and the reader is encouraged to watch the literature for documentation of inter-rater reliability and instrument validity.

Systematic Assessment of the Infant at the Breast

The Systematic Assessment of the Infant at the Breast (SAIB) tool was designed for use in the immediate postpartum period (Shrago & Bocar, 1990). The SAIB focuses on the assessment of the baby at the breast: aligning the infant at the breast; grasp and compression of the areolar tissue; and the use of swallowing as an indicator of intake. This tool is useful as a reminder of the success indicators for correct latch-on and positioning. The SAIB does not cover readiness cues in the infant or signs of feeding adequacy. See Table 1C–7 for the description of this tool.

Mother–Baby Assessment

The Mother–Baby Assessment (MBA) tool, although not as specific as the SAIB in its description of alignment, areolar grasp, and areolar compression, does cover readiness cues and feeding adequacy (Mulford, 1992). It also includes the mother in the assessment and gives a systematic method for scoring an early breastfeeding—much like Apgar scoring, which assigns a 1 or 2 for five aspects of the infant's physical condition following birth (color, heart rate, respiration, muscle tone, response to stimuli). See Table 1C–8 for a description of the MBA and Figure 1C–6 for a sample of the actual tool.

Infant Breastfeeding Assessment Tool

The Infant Breastfeeding Assessment Tool (IBFAT) was developed to assess the infant in the first few days after birth (Matthews, 1988). It assesses infant readiness for feeding, rooting, latching, and sucking behaviors. It is designed to be a cooperative effort between the mother and the health professional working with her. The last item on the tool relates to the mother's satisfaction with the feeding. Items 1

Table 1C–7   Systematic Assessment of the Infant at Breast

1. ALIGNMENT

Infant is in flexed position, relaxed and with no muscular rigidity. Infant's head and body are at breast level. Infant's head is aligned with trunk and is not turned laterally, hyperextended, or hyperflexed. Correct alignment of infant's body is confirmed by an imaginary line from ear to shoulder to iliac crest. Mother's breast is supported with cupped hand during first two weeks of breastfeeding.

2. AREOLAR GRASP

Mouth is open widely; lips are not pursed. Lips are visible and flanged outward. Complete seal and strong vacuum are formed by infant's mouth. Tongue covers lower alveolar ridge and is troughed (curved) around and below areola. No clicking or smacking sounds are heard during sucking. No drawing in (dimpling) of cheek pad is observed during sucking.

3. AREOLAR COMPRESSION

Mandible moves in a rhythmic motion. If indicated, a digital suck assessment reveals a wavelike motion of the tongue from the anterior mouth toward the oropharynx (a digital suck assessment is not routinely performed).

4. AUDIBLE SWALLOWING

Quiet sound of swallowing is heard. May be preceded by several sucking motions. May increase in frequency and consistency after milk ejection reflex occurs.

Source: Shrago, LC, Bocar, DL (1990). The infant's contribution to breastfeeding. *JOGNN*, 19:211, © AWHONN. Reprinted with permission of Lippincott-Raven Publishers.

Table 1C–8 The Mother–Baby Assessment for Breastfeeding

1. SIGNALING

- Mother watches and listens for baby's cues. She may hold, stroke, rock, talk to baby. She stimulates baby if he is sleepy, calms baby if he is fussy.
- Baby gives readiness cues: stirring, alertness, rooting, sucking, hand-to-mouth, vocal cues, cry.

2. POSITIONING

- Mother holds baby in good alignment within latch-on range of nipple. Baby's body is slightly flexed, entire ventral surface facing mother's body. Baby's head and shoulders are supported.
- Baby roots well at breast, opens mouth wide, tongue cupped and covering lower gum.

3. FIXING

- Mother holds her breast to assist baby as needed, brings baby in close when his mouth is wide open. She may express drops of milk.
- Baby latches-on, takes all of nipple and about 2 cm (1 inch) of areola into mouth, then sucks, demonstrating recurrent burst–pause pattern.

4. MILK TRANSFER

- Mother reports feeling any of the following: thirst, uterine cramps, increased lochia, breast ache or tingling, relaxation, sleepiness. Milk leaks from opposite breast.
- Baby swallows audibly; milk is observed in baby's mouth; baby may spit up milk when burping. Rapid "call up sucking" rate (two sucks/second) changes to "nutritive sucking" rate of about 1 suck/second.

5. ENDING

- Mother's breasts are comfortable; she lets baby suck until he is finished. After nursing, her breasts feel softer; she has no lumps, engorgement, or nipple soreness.
- Baby releases breast spontaneously, appears satiated. Baby does not root when stimulated. Baby's face, arms, and hands are relaxed; baby may fall asleep.

Source: Mulford, C (1992). The mother–baby assessment (MBA): An "Apgar score" for breastfeeding. *J Hum Lact*, 8:79–82. Reprinted with permission of Human Sciences Press, Inc., and the author.

and 6 are not scored. Twelve is the highest score attainable. See Figures 1C–7 and 1C–8 for the actual IBFAT and the scoring graph.

Vancouver Breastfeeding Centre Assessment Guidelines

For mothers presented with problems, the Vancouver Breastfeeding Centre staff recommend following the process of assessment, analysis, diagnosis, intervention (care and counsel), and evaluation (Ellis, Livingstone, & Hewat, 1993).

Assessment—Focuses on behaviors and factors relevant to the expressed problem and breastfeeding kinetics.

Analysis—Analyze the assessment data to determine factors influencing the problem.

Diagnosis—Formulate a diagnosis that states the concern/problem and the factors related to it.

Figure 1C–6

The Mother–Baby Assessment for Breastfeeding Sample

Source: Mulford, C (1992). The mother–baby assessment (MBA): An "Apgar score" for breastfeeding. *J Hum Lact*, 8: 79–82. Reprinted with permission.

	M	B	HELP
Signaling	x	x	
Positioning	x	x	
Fixing	x		
Milk Transfer			
Ending			

Total Score   5 (With Help)

This is an assessment method for rating the progress of a mother and baby who are learning to breastfeed.

For every step, each person—both mother and baby—should receive an *x* before either one can be scored on the following step. If the observer does not observe any of the designated indicators, score 0 for that person on that step. If help is needed at any step for either the mother or the baby, check *Help* for that step. This notation will not change the total score for mother and baby.

Intervention—Plan care and counsel that specifically address the stated causal or related factors or forces.

Evaluation—Evaluate the effectiveness of the care in bringing about change in the problem or concern. Revise care and counsel until breastfeeding goals are met.

Because lactation and breastfeeding processes are influenced by many factors, a model of breastfeeding kinetics detailing causative factors and direct interventions to the appropriate process may be helpful. Interventions developed for a particular mother's problem should be designed to enhance the process. See Figure 1C–9 for Livingstone's (1995) description of breastfeeding kinetics.

B-R-E-A-S-T Observation Form

The B-R-E-A-S-T observation form was developed to evaluate six elements (Armstrong, 1990):

- **B** – Body position
- **R** – Responses of baby and mother
- **E** – Emotional bonding
- **A** – Anatomy and condition of breast and nipple
- **S** – Sucking
- **T** – Time spent sucking

It was designed to help professionals learn how to observe a breastfeed, and it gives a checklist of favorable signs and possible indications of a problem for each element. The form does not diagnose every breastfeeding difficulty, but it helps to screen mothers who need more careful attention. The counselor should provide follow-up, including history taking and suck assessment, to any mother and baby who score rather low on this observation and any mother whose baby is not gaining weight adequately.

The time spent in actual breastfeeding is an important observation, especially if the mother tends to terminate every feed in less than three or four minutes. Babies

Figure 1C–7

Infant Breastfeeding Assessment Tool

Source: Matthews, MK (1988). Developing an instrument to assess infant breastfeeding behavior in the early neonatal period. *Midwifery*, 4(4), 154–165. Reprinted with permission of Churchill Livingstone and the author.

Check the answer which best describes the baby's feeding behaviors at this feed.

1. When you picked baby up to feed was he/she

(a) deeply asleep (eyes closed, no observable movement except breathing)	(b) drowsy	(c) quiet and alert	(d) crying
_____	_____	_____	_____

2. In order to get the baby to begin this feed, did you or the nurse have to

(a) just place the baby on the breast as no effort was needed	(b) use mild stimulation such as unbundling, patting, or burping	(c) unbundle baby; sit baby back and forward; rub baby's body or limbs vigorously at the beginning and during the feeding	(d) baby could not be aroused
3	2	1	0
_____	_____	_____	_____

3. Rooting (definition: at touch of nipple to cheek, baby's head turns toward the nipple, the mouth opens, and baby attempts to fix mouth on the nipple). When the baby was placed beside the breast, he/she

(a) rooted effectively at once	(b) needed some coaxing, prompting, or encouragement to root	(c) rooted poorly even with coaxing	(d) did not try to root
3	2	1	0
_____	_____	_____	_____

4. How long from placing baby at the breast does it take for the baby to latch-on and start to suck?

(a) starts to feed at once (0–3 min)	(b) 3 to 10 minutes	(c) over 10 minutes	(d) did not feed
3	2	1	0
_____	_____	_____	_____

5. Which of the following phrases best describes the baby's feeding pattern at this feed?

(a) baby did not suck	(b) sucked poorly; weak sucking; some sucking efforts for short periods	(c) sucked fairly well; sucked off and on, but needed encouragement	(d) sucked well throughout on one or both breasts
0	1	2	3
_____	_____	_____	_____

6. How do you feel about the way the baby fed at this feeding?

(a) very pleased	(b) pleased	(c) fairly pleased	(d) not pleased
_____	_____	_____	_____

who are given very abbreviated feeds may not be getting the fat-rich hindmilk, receiving instead more lactose-containing foremilk than they can easily digest. Some mothers terminate feeds before the milk-ejection reflex has moved the fat down the ducts to the lactiferous sinuses; they may have babies who fail to gain weight as a result.

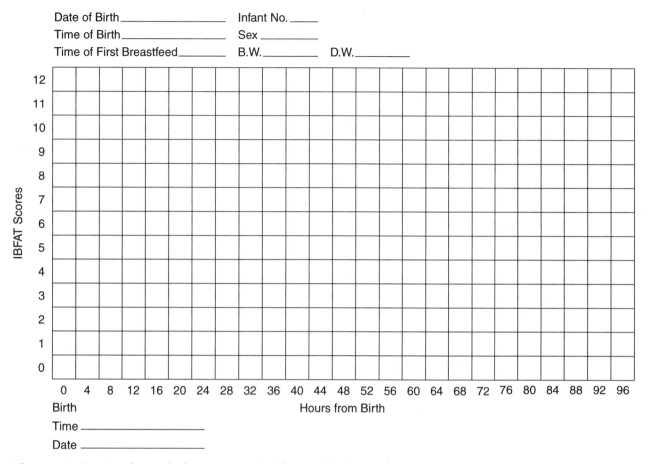

Date of Birth_____   Infant No._____
Time of Birth_____   Sex_____
Time of First Breastfeed_____   B.W._____   D.W._____

Figure 1C-8   Graph on which IBFAT is scored for each feeding

Source: Matthews, MK (1993). Assessments and suggested interventions to assist newborn breastfeeding behavior. *J Hum Lact*, 9:243–48. Reprinted with permission of Human Sciences Press, Inc., and author.

LATCH

One charting system developed to provide a systematic method for gathering information about individual breastfeeding sessions is the LATCH tool (Jensen, Wallace, & Kelsay, 1994). This system assigns a numerical value to five key components of breastfeeding. A 0, 1, or 2 is assigned to each component and a total score similar to an Apgar score is obtained. Using this system, the mother and infant can be assessed and definite areas needing intervention and teaching identified. See Figure 1C–10 for the scoring of these five key components.

DOCUMENTATION

Legal Issues

The legal implications of providing care to a mother and her baby where advice is offered or physical contact is made with either party must be recognized by lactation consultants, breastfeeding educators, and peer counselors. Guidelines to

Figure 1C–9

Breastfeeding kinetics

Source: Livingstone, V (1995). Breastfeeding kinetics: A problem-solving approach to breastfeeding difficulties. In: Simopoulos, AP, Dutra de Oliveira, JE, Desai, ID (Eds), Behavioral and Metabolic Aspects of Breastfeeding, *World Rev Nutr Diet*, 78:28–54. Basel: Karger. Reprinted with permission of Canadian Family Physician, Mississauga, Ontario, and the author. Modified from Livingstone, V (1990). Problem-solving formula for failure to thrive in breastfed infants. *Can Fam Phys*, 36:1541–45.

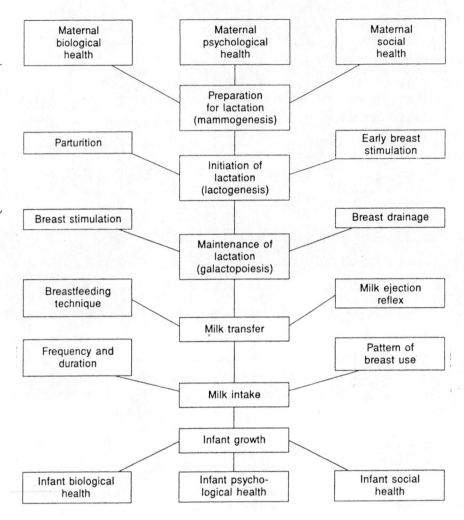

follow to minimize the risk of legal action include obtaining permission (definitely verbal; preferably written) before touching the client or infant, maintaining confidentiality, providing all services promised, and avoiding emotional stress in the client or family as a result of careless actions or choice of words. It is wise for the practitioner to check out the professional liability coverage of the institution where he or she is employed. For one who is self-employed or works as a consultant, liability coverage is essential.

Charting

Regardless of the counselor's work setting (hospital, public health agency, private doctor's office, private practice), documentation of each contact with a client is essential. Charting can be narrative or problem-oriented, such as the subjective, objective assessment plan (SOAP) or FOCUS note formats. Since the mother and infant usually have separate charts, counselors may have to document contact in both.

Clinical care plans are required for each patient by the Joint Commission on Accreditation of Healthcare Organizations. Public health agencies (like the USDA) also require breastfeeding encounters by staff to be documented in the patient's public health medical record.

Figure 1C–10

The LATCH scoring table

Source: Jenson, D, Wallace, S, Kelsay, P (1994). LATCH: A breastfeeding charting system and documentation tool. *JOGNN*, 23(1):29. Reprinted with permission of Lippincott-Raven Publishers and authors.

	0	1	2
L Latch	Too sleepy or reluctant No sustained latch or suck achieved	Repeated attempts for sustained latch or suck Hold nipple in mouth Stimulate to suck	Grasps breast Tongue down Lips flanged Rhythmical sucking
A Audible swallowing	None	A few with stimulation	Spontaneous and intermittent <24 hours old Spontaneous and frequent >24 hours old
T Type of nipple	Inverted	Flat	Everted (after stimulation)
C Comfort (breast/nipple)	Engorged Cracked, bleeding, large blisters, or bruises Severe discomfort	Filling Reddened/small blisters or bruises Mild/moderate discomfort	Soft Nontender
H Hold (positioning)	Full assist (staff holds infant at breast)	Minimal assist (i.e., elevate head of bed; place pillows for support) Teach one side; mother does other Staff holds and then mother takes over	No assist from staff Mother able to position and hold infant

Traditional methods of charting (good, fair, poor) are subjective and imprecise and do not communicate concrete information to other staff caring for the mother and infant. Charting a breastfeeding session should cover, at a minimum, whether the infant accomplished areolar grasp and whether there was evidence of milk transfer. It should also contain information on the infant's state (hydrated versus dehydrated, weight loss or gain, presence of hyperbilirubinemia, hypoglycemia, etc.) and the mother's state (breasts—soft, full, engorged; nipples—no trauma noted, color changes, skin integrity; presence of uterine contractions; increased lochia flow, etc). The mother's emotional state and her comprehension of any recommendations made are also important to note in the medical record. Plans for follow-up should be realistic, achievable, and implemented in a timely manner. Referrals made should be documented, and written instructions provided to the mother.

POST-TEST

For questions 1 to 4, choose the best answer from the following key:

   A. Nonnutritive sucking   C. Swallowing

   B. Sucking and swallowing   D. Sucking, swallowing, and breathing

1. _____ occurs between expiration and inspiration.

2. _____ increases peristalsis and enhances digestive fluid secretion.

3. _____ is established by 32 weeks gestational age.

4. _____ is well coordinated by 37 weeks gestational age.

For questions 5 to 8, choose the best answer.

5. Buccal fat pads

   A. are located between the temporalis and buccinator muscles.

   B. contribute toward the establishment of positive pressure in the infant's oral cavity during sucking.

   C. are layers of fat in ligaments.

   D. provide stability during feeding.

6. Breastmilk stool

   A. has a high pH, which discourages replication of enteropathogens.

   B. is scant and occasional in the exclusively breastfed neonate.

   C. changes in color, consistency, and frequency as the infant ages.

   D. is present after every breastfeeding in all babies exclusively breastfed for six months.

7. Urine output

   A. is always an indication of adequate intake.

   B. increases after the transitional milk appears.

   C. should be at least four wet diapers per 24 hours.

   D. will be concentrated and scant in the first month.

8. Symptoms of appetite spurts include generalized fussiness in an infant who has previously been content after feedings and

   A. decreased feeding frequency and increased feeding duration.

   B. increased feeding frequency and decreased feeding duration.

   C. decreased feeding frequency and decreased feeding duration.

   D. increased feeding frequency and increased feeding duration.

For questions 9 to 12, choose the best answer from the following key:

   A. Drowsiness and increased uterine contractions

   B. Insufficient milk supply

   C. Swallowing and satisfaction after a feed

   D. Color, opaqueness, creaminess of milk

9. Concern of mother that often undermines breastfeeding success.

10. Infant indicator of a good feed.

11. Not related to the adequacy of the milk supply.

12. Maternal indicator of a good feed.

For questions 13 to 16, choose the best answer.

13. All of the following can assist the breastfeeding assessment except:
    A. visual inspection of breast appearance while infant is feeding.
    B. position of the baby's head.
    C. amount of time the infant's eyes are open versus closed.
    D. presence or absence of nipple pain.

14. Which describes the action of the tongue in removing milk from the breast?
    A. Smacking
    B. Draining
    C. Stripping
    D. Tasting

15. Which describes the sucking pattern at the start of a feed and after the first milk-ejection reflex?
    A. Long bursts of sucking and long pauses
    B. Long bursts of sucking and short pauses
    C. Short bursts of sucking and long pauses
    D. Short bursts of sucking and short pauses

16. Sucking problems can be caused by all of the following except:
    A. neuromotor–neuroendocrine dysfunction.
    B. anatomic variation in infant's oral cavity.
    C. early introduction of artificial teats.
    D. birth by cesarean section.

For questions 17 to 20, choose the best answer from the following key:
    A. Large amounts of IV fluid with high dextrose concentrations given to mother during labor
    B. Use of nipple shields
    C. Pathological engorgement
    D. Milk inspissation

17. Clouds the calculation of birth weight and initial weight loss in baby.

18. Increased breastmilk thickness or decreased fluidity secondary to fluid absorption.

19. Reduces stimulation to the nipple and areola.

20. Leads to pressure atrophy of the alveoli.

References

Alexander, JM, Grant, AM, Campbell, MJ (1993). Randomized control trial of breast shells and Hoffman's exercises for inverted and non-protractile nipples. *Br Med J*, 304:1030-32.

Amatayakul, K, Vutyavanich, T, Tanthayaphinant, O, Tovanabutra, S, Yupadee, Y, Drewett, RF (1987). Serum prolactin and cortisol levels after sucking for varying periods of time and the effect of a nipple shield. *Acta Obstet Gynecol Scand*, 66:47-51.

Amiel-Tison, C (1967). Neurological evaluation of the maturity of newborn infant. *Arch Dis Child*, 43:89-93.

Anderson, GC (1991). Current knowledge about skin-to-skin (kangaroo) care for preterm infants. *J Perinatol*, 11(3):216-26.

Ardran, GM, Kemp, FH, Lind, J (1958). A cineradiographic study of breastfeeding. *Br J Radiol*, 31:156-62.

Armstrong, HC (1990). *Lactation Management Topic Outlines*. Nairobi, Kenya: IBFAN Africa.

Auerbach, KG (1990). Breastfeeding fallacies: Their relationship to understanding lactation. *Birth*, 17(1):44-49.

Auerbach, KG, Eggert, LD (1987). The importance of infant sucking patterns when a breast-fed baby fails to thrive. *J Trop Pediatr*, 33(3):156-57.

Bocar, DL (1993). *Breastfeeding Educator Program*, pp. 50, 59, 67, 73, 78, 115, 150. Lactation Consultant Services, Oklahoma City.

Bocar, DL, Shrago, L (1993). Breastfeeding education. In: Riordan, J, Auerbach, K (Eds), *Breastfeeding and Human Lactation*, pp. 181-214. Boston: Jones and Bartlett.

Bosma, J, Showacre, J (1975). Development of upper respiratory anatomy and function. Rockville, MD: U.S. Dept. Of Health, Education and Welfare.

Bowen-Jones, A, Thompson, C, Drewett, RF (1982). Milk flow and sucking rates during breastfeeding. *Dev Med Child Neuro*, 24:626-33.

Bu'lock, F, Woolridge, MW, Baum, JD (1990). Development of coordination of sucking, swallowing and breathing: Ultrasound study of term and preterm infants. *Dev Med Child Neurol*, 32:669-78.

Craig, HR (1993). *Lactational Insufficiency and Induced Lactation*. Presentation at International Lactation Consultants Association annual meeting, Scottsdale, AZ.

Daly, S, Owens, R, Hartman, P (1993). The short-term synthesis and infant-regulated removal of milk in lactating women. *Exp Physiol*, 78:209-20.

deCoopman, JD (1993). Breastfeeding after pituitary resection: Support for a theory of autocrine control of milk supply? *J Hum Lact*, 9(1):35-40.

East Central Health District (1993). Prenatal Survey Tool. Augusta, GA.

Eiger, MS, Olds, SW (1987). *The Complete Book of Breastfeeding*. New York: Workman.

Ellis, D (1986). Supporting the breast-feeding dad. *Can Fam Physician*, 32:541-45.

Ellis, DJ, Livingstone, VH, Hewat, RJ (1993). Assisting the breastfeeding mother: A problem-solving process. *J Hum Lact*, 9:89-93.

Eppink, H (1969). An experiment to determine a basis for nursing decisions in regard to time of initiation of breastfeeding. *Nurs Res*, 18(4):292-99.

Ezzo, G, Bucknam, R (1995). *On Becoming Baby Wise*. Sisters, OR: Multnomah Books.

Frantz, AG, Kleinberg, DL, Noel, GL (1972). Studies on prolactin in man. *Rec Prog Hor Res*, 28:527-90.

Hales, DJ (1981). Promoting breastfeeding: Strategies for changing hospital policy. *Stud Fam Plan*, 12:167-72.

Herbst, JJ (1981). Development of suck and swallowing. In: Lebenthal, E (Ed), *Textbook of gastroenterology and nutrition in infancy*, Vol. 1, pp. 97-107. New York: Plenum Press.

Horne, HW, Scott, JM (1969). Intrauterine contraceptive devices in women with proven fertility: A five-year follow-up study. *Fertil Steril*, 20(3):400-4.

Huggins, K (1990). *The Nursing Mother's Companion*, p. 26. Boston: Harvard Common Press.

Jackson, DA, Woolridge, MW, Imong, SM, McLeod, CN, Yotabootr, Y, Wongsawat, L, Amatayakul, K, Baum, JD (1987). The automatic sampling shield: A device for sampling suckled breastmilk. *Early Hum Dev,* 15:295-306.

Jenson, D, Wallace, S, Kelsay, P (1994). LATCH: A breastfeeding charting system and documentation tool. *JOGNN,* 23:27-32.

Kaitz, M, Lapidot, P, Bronner, R, Eidelman, AL (1992). Parturient women can recognize their infants by touch. *Dev Psychol,* 28:35-39.

Keepler, AB (1988). The use of intravenous fluids during labor. *Birth,* 15:75-79.

Kesaree, N, Banapurmath, CR, Banapurmath, S, Shamanur, K (1993). Treatment of inverted nipples using a disposable syringe. *J Hum Lact,* 9(1):27-29.

King, FS (1992). *Helping Mothers to Breastfeed.* Nairobi, Kenya: African Medical and Research Foundation.

Lawrence, RA (1989). *Breastfeeding: A Guide for the Medical Profession,* 3rd ed. St. Louis: Mosby.

Livingstone, VL (1995). Breastfeeding kinetics: A problem-solving approach to breastfeeding difficulties. In: Simopoulos, AP, Dutra de Oliveira, JE, Desai, ID (Eds), Behavioral and metabolic aspects of breastfeeding. *World Rev Nutr Diet,* 78:28-54. Basel: Karger.

Maher, SM (1988). *An Overview of Solutions to Breastfeeding and Sucking Problems.* Franklin Park, IL: La Leche League International.

Marmet, C, Shell, E (1984). Training neonates to suck correctly. *MCN,* 9(6):401-7.

Marmet, C, Shell, E (1986). *Lactation Forms: A Guide to Lactation Consultant Charting.* Encino, CA: The Lactation Institute.

Mathew, OP, Bhatia, J (1989). Sucking and breathing patterns during breast and bottle feeding in term neonates. *Am J Dis Child,* 143:588-92.

Matthews, MK (1988). Developing an instrument to assess infant breastfeeding behavior in the early neonatal period. *Midwifery,* 4(4):154-65.

Matthews, MK (1993). Assessment and suggested interventions to assist newborn breastfeeding behavior. *J Hum Lact,* 9(4):243-48.

McBride, MC, Danner, SC (1987). Sucking disorders in neurologically impaired infants. *Clin Perinatol,* 14:109-30.

Measel, CP, Anderson, GC (1979). Nonnutritive sucking during tube feedings: Effect on clinical course in premature infants. *JOGNN,* 8:265-72.

Miller, AJ (1982). Deglutition. *Physiol Rev,* 62:129-83.

Minchin, MK (1989a). *Breastfeeding Matters: What We Need to Know about Infant Feeding.* Victoria, Australia: George Allen Unwin & Alma.

Minchin, MK (1989b). Positioning for breastfeeding. *Birth,* 16(2):67-80.

Mohrbacher, N, Stock, J (1991). *The Breastfeeding Answer Book.* Franklin Park, IL: La Leche League International.

Morris, SE, Klein, MD (1987). *Pre-Feeding Skills.* Tucson: Therapy Skill Builders.

Mulford, C (1992). The mother–baby assessment (MBA): An "Apgar score" for breastfeeding. *J Hum Lact,* 8:79-82.

Neifert, MR, Seacat, JM (1985). Contemporary breastfeeding management. *Clin Perinatol,* 12(2):319-42.

Riordan, J, Auerbach, KG (1993). *Breastfeeding and Human Lactation.* Boston: Jones and Bartlett.

Rodenstein, DO, Perimutter, N, Stanescu, DC (1985). Infants are not obligatory nose breathers. *Am Rev Respir Dis,* 131:343-47.

Ross, M (1987). *Back to the Breast: Retraining Infant Sucking Patterns.* Lactation Consultant Series, Unit 15. Garden City Park, NY: Avery.

Shrago, LC, Bocar, DL (1990). The infant's contribution to breastfeeding. *JOGNN,* 19:209-15.

Weaver, LT, Ewing, G, Taylor, LC (1988). The bowel habits of milk-fed infants. *J Pediatr Gastroenterol Nutr,* 7(4):568-71.

Weber, F, Woolridge, MW, Baum, JD (1986). An ultrasonographic study of the organization of sucking and swallowing by newborn infants. *Dev Med Child Neurol,* 28:19-24.

Weichert, EE (1980). Prolactin cycling and the management of breastfeeding failure. *Adv Pediatr,* 27:391-407.

Widstrom, AM, Ransjo-Arvidson, AB, Christensson, K, Matthiesen, AS, Winberg, J, Uvnas-Moberg, K (1987). Gastric suction in healthy newborn infants: Effects on circulation and developing feeding behavior. *Acta Paediatr Scand,* 76(4):566-72.

Wolff, PH (1968). The serial organization of sucking in the young infant. *Pediatrics,* 42:943-56.

Woolridge, MW (1986). The 'anatomy' of infant sucking. *Midwifery,* 2:164-71.

Ziemer, M, Pigeon, JG (1993). Skin changes and pain in the nipple during the first week of lactation. *JOGNN,* 22:247-56.

ADDITIONAL READINGS

Anderson, GC, McBride, MR, Dahm, J, Ellis, MK, Vidyasagar, D (1982). Development of sucking in term infants from birth to four hours postbirth. *Res Nurs Health,* 5(1):21-27.

Arizona Healthy Mothers, Healthy Babies Breastfeeding Task Force (1989). *Model Breastfeeding Hospital Policy and Breastfeeding Education Protocol.* Arizona Department of Health Services, Office of Nutrition.

Auerbach, KG (1988). Beyond the issue of accuracy: Evaluating patient education materials for breastfeeding mothers. *J Hum Lact,* 4:108-10.

Auerbach, KG, Gartner, L (1987). Breastfeeding and human milk: Their association with jaundice in the neonate. *Clin Perinatol,* 14:89-107

Barr, RG, Kramer, MS, Pless, IB, Boisjoly, C, Ledye, D (1989). Feeding and temperament as determinants of early infant crying/fussing behavior. *Pediatrics,* 84:514-21.

Barr, RG, Elias, NF (1988). Nursing interval and maternal responsivity: Effect on early infant crying. *Pediatrics,* 81(4):529-36.

Beller, F (1990). Development and anatomy of the breast. In: Mitchell, GW, Bassett, LW (Eds), *The Female Breast and Its Disorders* (pp. 1-12). Baltimore: Williams & Wilkins.

Blass, EM, Teicher, MH (1980). Sucking. *Science*, 210:15-22.

Bloom, K, Goldbloom, RB, Robinson, SC, Stevens, FE (1982). Breast versus formula feeding. *Acta Paediatr Scand* (Supp), 300:1-26.

Bocar, D, Moore, K (1987). *Acquiring the Parental Role: A Theoretical Perspective*. Lactation Consultant Series, Unit 16. Garden City Park, NY: Avery.

Bocar, DL, Shrago, LC (1989). Pre-discharge breastfeeding assessment. *Breastfeeding Abst*, 9(1):1-2.

Bottorff, JL (1989). Persistence in breastfeeding: a phenomenological investigation. *J Adv Nurs*, 15:201-9.

Brazelton, TB (1986). *Infants and Mothers: Differences in Development*. New York: Dell.

Brillinger, MF (1990). Helping adults learn. *J Hum Lact*, 6(4):171-75.

Bryant, C, Roy, M (1989). *Best Start Training Manual*. Tampa: Best Start.

Cernoch, JM, Porter, RH (1985). Recognition of maternal axillary odors by infants. *Child Dev*, 56:1593-98.

Coreil, J, Murphy, J (1988). Maternal commitment, lactation practices, and breastfeeding duration. *JOGNN*, 17:273-78.

Cortial, C, Lezine, I (1974). Comparative study of nutritive sucking in the newborn (premature and full-term). *Early Child Dev Care*, 3:221-28.

Dahl, M, Sundelin, C (1986). Early feeding problems in an affluent society. Part 2: Determinants. *Acta Paediatr Scand*, 74:380-87.

DeCarvalho, M, Robertson, S, & Klaus, MH (1984). Does the duration and frequency of early breastfeeding affect nipple pain? *Birth*, 11:81-84.

DeCasper, AJ, Fifer, WP (1980). Of human bonding: Newborns prefer their mothers' voices. *Science*, 208:1174-76.

DeChateau, P, Holmberg, H, Jakobson, K, Einberg, J (1977). A study of factors promoting and inhibiting lactation. *Dev Med Child Neurol*, 19:575-84.

Dewey, K, Lonnerdal, B (1986). Infant self-regulation of breast-milk intake. *Acta Paediatr Scand*, 75:893-98.

Dodgson, J (1989). Early identification of potential breastfeeding problems. *J Hum Lact*, 5:80-81.

Drewett, RF, Woolridge, MW (1979). Sucking patterns of human babies on the breast. *Early Human Develop*, 3(4):315-20.

Ekwo, EE, Dusdieker, L, Booth, B, Seals, B (1984). Psychosocial factors influencing the duration of breastfeeding by primigravidas. *Acta Paediatr Scand*, 73:241-47.

Emde, R (1975). Human wakefulness and biological rhythms after birth. *Arch Gen Psychiatry*, 32:780-83.

Escott, R (1989). Positioning, attachment and milk transfer. *Breastfeeding Rev*, 14:31-37.

Feinstein, JM, Berkelhamer, JE, Gruszka, ME, Wang, CA, Carey, AE (1986). Factors related to early termination of breast-feeding in an urban population. *Pediatrics*, 78:21-25.

Ferris, AM, McCabe, LT, Allen, LH, Pelto, GH (1987). Biological and sociocultural determinants of successful lactation among women in eastern Connecticut. *J Am Diet Assoc*, 87:316-21.

Frantz, K (1991). Keep breastfeeding simple, keep it easy, keep it fun. *Birth*, 18(4):228-29.

Freed, GL, Lander, S, Schanler, RJ (1991). A practical guide to successful breast-feeding management. *AJDC*, 145: 917-21.

Friesen, HG, Cowden, EA (1989). Lactation and galactorrhea. In: DeGroot, LJ (Ed), *Endocrinology in Pregnancy*, pp. 274-86. Philadelphia: WB Saunders.

Goodine, LA, Fried, PA (1984). Infant feeding practices: Pre- and postnatal factors affecting choice of method and the duration of breastfeeding. *Can J Pub Health*, 75:439-44.

Graef, P, McGhee, K, Rozycki, J, Fascina-Jones, D, Clark, JA, Thompson, J, Brooten, D (1988). Postpartum concerns of breastfeeding mothers. *J Nurse-Midwifery*, 33(2):62-66.

Hill, PD, Humenick, SS (1989). Unsufficient milk supply. *J Nurs Scholar*, 21(3):145-58.

Hoffmann, JB (1953). A suggested treatment for inverted nipples. *Am J Obstet Gynecol*, 66:346.

Humenick, S, Van Steenkiste, S (1983). Early indicators of breast-feeding progress. *Iss Compr Pediatr Nurs*, 6:205-15.

Institute of Medicine (IOM) (1991). *Nutrition during lactation*. Washington, DC: National Academy Press.

Jain, L, Sivieri, E, Bhutani, VK (1987). Energetics and mechanics of nutritive sucking in the preterm and term neonate. *J Pediatr*, 11:894-98.

Jenks, M (1991). Latch assessment in the hospital nursery. *J Hum Lact*, 7:19-20.

Kearney, MH, Cronenwett, LR, Barrett, JA (1990). Breastfeeding problems in the first week postpartum. *Nurs Res*, 39(2).

Lau, C, Henning, SJ (1989). A noninvasive method for determining patterns of milk intake in the breast-fed infant. *J Pediatr Gastroenterol Nutr*, 9:481-87.

Livingstone, VL (1990). Problem-solving formula for failure to thrive in breastfed infants. *Can Fam Phys*, 36: 1541-45.

Loughlin, H (1985). Early termination of breast-feeding: Identifying those at risk. *Pediatrics*, 75:508-13.

Lovelady, CA, Lonnerdal, B, Dewey, KG (1990). Lactation performance of exercising women. *Am J Clin Nutr*. 52(1):103-9.

Makin, CW, Porter, RH (1989). Attractiveness of latching females' breast odors to neonates. *Child Dev*, 60:803-910.

Matthews, MK (1991a). Mothers' satisfaction with their neonates' breastfeeding behavior in the early neonatal period. *Midwifery*, 4(4):154-65.

Matthews, MK (1991b). Mothers' satisfaction with their neonates' breastfeeding behaviors. *JOGNN*, 20:49-55.

Mills, AF (1990). Surveillance for anemia: Risk factors in patterns of milk intake. *Arch Dis Child*, 65(4):428-31.

Morgan, J (1986). A study of mothers' breastfeeding concerns. *Birth*, 13(2):104-8.

Morton, JA (1992). Ineffective sucking: A possible consequence of obstructive positioning. *J Hum Lact*, 8(2): 79-82.

Mulford, C (1990). Subtle signs and symptoms of the letdown reflex. *J Hum Lact*, 6:177-78.

Neifert, MR, Seacat, JM (1986). A guide to successful breastfeeding. *Contemp Pediatr*, 3:1-26.

Newman, J (1990). Breastfeeding problems associated with the early introduction of bottles and pacifiers. *J Hum Lact*, 6:59-63.

Neyzi, O, Gulecyuz, M, Dincer, Z, Olgun, P, Kutluay, T, Uzel, N, Saner, G (1991). An educational intervention on promotion of breastfeeding complemented by continuing support. *Paediatr Perinatal Epidemol*, 5: 299-303.

Nicolaides, N (1974). Skin lipids: Their biochemical uniqueness. *Science*, 186:19-26.

Osborne, MP (1991). Breast development and anatomy. In: Harris, JR, Hellman, S, Henderson, IC, Kinne, DW (Eds), *Breast Diseases*. Philadelphia: JB Lippincott.

Page-Goertz, S (1989). Discharge planning for the breastfeeding dyad. *Pediatr Nurs*, 15(5):543-44.

Porter, RH, Makin, JW, Davis, LB, Christensen, KM (1991). An assessment of the salient olfactory environment of formula-fed infants. *Physiology Behavior*, 50:907-11.

Prechtl, HFR (1974). The behavioral states of the newborn infant (review). *Brain Res*, 76:185-212.

Pridham, KF (1993). Anticipatory guidance of parents of new infants: Potential contribution of the internal working model construct. *Image*, 25:49-56.

Redman, BK (1988). *The Process of Patient Education*, 6th ed. St. Louis: Mosby.

Renfrew, M (1989). Positioning the baby at the breast: More than a visual skill. *J Hum Lact*, 5:13-15.

Renfrew, M, Fisher, C, Arms, S (1990). *Breastfeeding: Getting Breastfeeding Right for You*. Berkeley, CA: Celestial Arts.

Rentschler, DD (1991). Correlates of successful breastfeeding. *Image J Nurs Sch*, 23:151-54.

Righard, L, Alade, MO (1992). Sucking technique and its effect on success of breastfeeding. *Birth*, 19:185-89.

Riordan, J (1985). Readable, relevant, reliable: The three "R's" of breastfeeding pamphlets. *Breastfeeding Abst*, 5:5-6.

Riordan, J, Countryman, BA (1980). Basics of breastfeeding. Part IV: Preparation for breastfeeding and early optimal functioning. *JOGNN*, 9:273-83.

Rowe, L, Cumming, F, King, R, Mackey, C (1992). A comparison of two methods of breastfeeding management. *Austr Fam Phys*, 21:286-94.

Rush, JP, Kitch, TL (1991). A randomized, controlled trial to measure the frequency of use of a hospital telephone line for new parents. *Birth*, 18:193-97.

Russell, MJ (1976). Human olfactory communication. *Nature*, 260:520-22.

Salariya, E, Easton, PM, Cater, JI (1978). Duration of breastfeeding after early initiation and frequent feeding. *Lancet*, 2:1141-43.

Shrago, LC (1992). The breastfeeding dyad: Early assessment, documentation, and interventions. *NAACOG's Clinical Issues Perinatal Women's Health*, 3:583-97.

Simon, JL, Johnson, CA, Liese, BS (1988). A family practice "breastfeeding hotline": Description and preliminary results. *Fam Med*, 20:224-26.

Smith, WL, Erenberg, A, Nowak, A (1985). Physiology of sucking in the normal term infant using real-time ultrasound. *Radiology*, 156:379-81.

Smith, WL, Erenberg, A, Nowak, A (1988). Imaging evaluation of the human nipple during breast-feeding. *Am J Dis Child*, 142(1):76-78.

Taylor, PM, Maloni, JA, Brown, DR (1986). Early sucking and prolonged breast-feeding. *Am J Dis Child*, 140:151-54.

Taylor, PM, Maloni, JA, Taylor, FH, Campbell, SB (1985). Extra early mother–infant contact and duration of breast-feeding. *Acta Paediatr Scand*, 316(Suppl):15-22.

Verronen, P (1982). Breastfeeding: Reasons for giving up and transient lactational crisis. *Acta Paediatr Scand*, 71:447-50.

Vigliani, MB (1991). Antenatal lactation—a link with preterm labor. *S Afr Med J*, 80(8):410.

Walker, M (1989). Functional assessment of infant breastfeeding patterns. *Birth*, 16(3):140-46.

Walker, M (1989). Management of selected early breastfeeding problems seen in clinical practice. *Birth*, 16: 148-58.

Williams, JL (1985). Assessment and stabilization of the newborn. In: Daze, AM, Scanlon, J (Eds.), *Neonatal Nursing*, pp. 18-24. Baltimore: University Park Press.

Winikoff, B, LauKaran, VH, Myers, D, Stone, R (1986). Dynamics of infant feeding: Mother, professionals, and the institutional context in a large urban hospital. *Pediatrics*, 77:357-65.

Woolridge, MW, Baum, JD (1987). Ultrasonic study of sucking and swallowing by newborn infants (letter). *Dev Med Child Neurol*, 29(1):121-22.

Woolridge, MW, Ingram, JC, Baum, JD (1990). Do changes in pattern of breast usage alter the baby's nutrient intake? *Lancet*, 336:395-97.

Wright, A (1983). Prediction of duration of breastfeeding. *J Epidemiol Comm Health*, 37:89-91.

CHAPTER 2

Common Problems in Breastfeeding

SECTION A

Areolar and Nipple Tissue Structural Elements and Wound Healing

Jan B. Simpson, RN, BSN, IBCLC

LEARNING OBJECTIVES

At the completion of this section, the learner will be able to do the following:

1. Identify the epidermis and dermis layers of skin and discuss their functions.
2. Discuss the role of keratin in relation to the breast.
3. Discuss the roles of the sebaceous gland and sebum in relation to the breast and breastfeeding.
4. Discuss the role of tissue repair: dry wound healing versus moist wound healing.
5. Discuss the role nutrition plays in wound healing.

OUTLINE

  I. Skin

    A. Epidermis

    B. Keratin

    C. Dermis

  II. Sebaceous Glands

    A. Sebum

III. Tissue Repair

    A. Dry wound healing

    B. Moist wound healing

IV. Nutrition and Wound Healing

PRE-TEST

For questions 1 to 4, choose the single best answer.

1. The skin's functions include
    A. protective covering.
    B. respiratory functions.
    C. excretory functions.
    D. All of the above.

2. _____ is a layer of protein accumulated on the epidermis layer of the skin.
    A. Sebum
    B. Keratin
    C. Galactorrhea
    D. Lactoprotein

3. The epidermis layer is composed of
    A. stratified dermis.
    B. blood vessels that nourish all of the skin.
    C. stratified squamous epithelium.
    D. dermal nerve fibers.

4. The dermis layer is composed of
    A. fibrous connective tissue.
    B. stratified squamous epithelium.
    C. keratin.
    D. lactodermis fibers.

For questions 5 to 12, choose the best answer from the following key:

    A. epidermis   **D. sebum**
    B. dermis   **E. sebaceous glands**
    C. keratin

5. Montgomery's tubercles are _____.

6. _____ is bacteriostatic and fungicidal and contains enzymes like lysozyme that break down bacterial cells.

7. The cells of _____ accumulate, become hardened, and die, creating a covering of a tough protective substance that prevents the escape of water from underlying tissues and the entry of various microorganisms.

8. _____ is consistently sloughed off and replaced with a new layer, which enables the body to clean itself of adherent microorganisms.

9. _____ assists in protecting the nipple and areola during sucking and also maintains an acid pH on the areola.

10. _____ protects underlying tissues against water loss and damage.

11. _____ protects the underlying epithelial cells from wear and tear.

12. _____ accommodates the blood vessels that nourish all of the skin cells.

For questions 13 to 16, choose the best answer.

13. _____ is the replacement of dead or damaged cells by new healthy cells.
    A. Tissue repair
    B. Epithelial migration
    C. Regenerative epithelial repair
    D. All of the above.

14. In most nipple abrasions, the tissue that is lost is the superficial layer of the
    A. dermis.
    B. keratin.
    C. epidermis.
    D. subcutaneous layer.

15. In most nipple abrasions, the healing process that occurs is
    A. the acceleration of the normal process of basal cell maturation.
    B. epithelial regenerative repair.
    C. Both A and B.
    D. None of the above.

16. _____ may have a protective function for the rapid multiplication of basal cells and its fluid will be absorbed rapidly if left alone.
    A. Sebaceous gland
    B. Blister
    C. Lactiferous boil
    D. Montgomery's tubercle

For questions 17 to 20, choose the best answer from the following key:
    A. moist wound healing   **C. internal moisture**
    B. dry wound healing   **D. surface wetness**

17. _____ involves covering the wound to prevent air exposure and the application of a medium, which is permeable to water vapor and oxygen, so that an anaerobic environment is not produced at the wound surface and is not penetrable to bacteria.

18. Scab formation that occurs with _____ may present an impediment to the migration of epidermal cells across the surface of the wound during the healing process.

19. The retaining of _____ is believed to assist in the closure and healing of a fissure without the formation of a scab.

20. _____ contributes to nipple tenderness and damage.

Skin

One of the many functions of skin is that of functioning as a protective covering. Respiratory functions of the skin include the production of sweat. Excretory functions include milk secretion. The skin is composed of two distinctive layers, called the epidermis and dermis, and a keratin layer that is located on the surface, which is sloughed off to help eliminate microscopic waste. See Module 3, *The Science of Breastfeeding,* Chapter 1, for more information on the anatomy and physiology of the breast.

EPIDERMIS

The *epidermis* is a layer that is composed of stratified squamous epithelium. The epidermis functions as a protection against water loss and damage for underlying tissues. Epidermal cells undergo keratinization as they are pushed toward the surface.

KERATIN

The epidermis accumulates a protein called *keratin*. As this transpires, the cells become hardened and die. This action creates a covering of a tough protective substance that prevents the escape of water from underlying tissues and the entry

Figure 2A–1

Skin layers.

Source: Lauwers, J, Woessner, C (1989). *Counseling the Nursing Mother,* p. 74. Garden City Park, NY: Avery Publishing Company. Reprinted with permission.

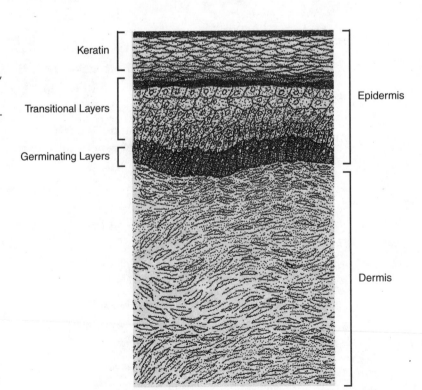

of various microorganisms. The production of epidermal cells is balanced with the velocity at which they are lost. Keratin is consistently sloughed off and replaced with a new layer, which enables the body to clean itself of adherent microorganisms. It also protects the underlying epithelial cells from wear and tear (Ham & Cormack, 1979; Hole, 1981; Wheater, Burkitt, & Daniels, 1979).

DERMIS

The epidermis is tightly bound to the second and deeper connective tissue of the skin called the *dermis*. It is a layer that is substantially composed of fibrous connective tissue that binds the epidermis to underlying tissues. It accommodates the blood vessels that nourish all of the skin cells, including those of the epidermis. Nerve tissue is distributed throughout the dermis layer. Various dermal nerve fibers convey impulses to muscles and glands of the skin (Figure 2A–1). Other dermal nerve fibers are associated with various sensory receptors in the skin (Hole, 1981; Wheater, Burkitt, & Daniels, 1979).

Sebaceous Glands

The skin surrounding the nipple, the areola, is pigmented and contains sebaceous glands, which hypertrophy and form papillae during pregnancy. These are referred to as Montgomery's tubercles and are not associated with hair follicles like other sebaceous glands of the body. Each sebaceous gland is a little sac with a lining of epithelial cells that proliferate and, by this process, more and more cells are forced into the interior of the sac. At the same time their cytoplasm becomes filled with a mixture of lipid material and cellular debris called sebum (Ham & Cormack, 1979; Hole, 1981; Wheater, Burkitt, & Daniels, 1979).

SEBUM

Sebum is produced by cells as they move from the wall toward the inside of the sac, where they die and break down. The sebum is then secreted by the gland, which lubricates the skin. Sebum is bacteriostatic and fungicidal and contains enzymes like lysozyme that break down bacterial cells. Sebum protects the nipple and areola during sucking and also maintains an acid pH on the areola (Ham & Cormack, 1979; Hole, 1981; Wheater, Burkitt, & Daniels, 1979).

Tissue Repair

Tissue repair is the replacement of dead or damaged cells by new healthy cells. If the damage of the tissue is shallow, epithelial cells along its border are prompted to reproduce quickly, and these new cells then fill in the break in the tissue. If the tissue injury is expanded to the dermis or subcutaneous layer, other tissues become implicated; and the repair process is more complicated. Hole (1981) described the healing process:

If normal skin (A) is injured deeply (B), (C) blood escapes from dermal blood vessels, and (D) a blood clot soon forms. The blood clot and dried tissue fluid form a scab (E) that protects the damaged region. Later, blood vessels send out branches, and fibroblasts migrate into the area (F). The fibroblasts produce new connective tissue fibers, and when the skin is largely repaired, the scab sloughs off (G) (see Figure 2A–2).

Repair of a large patch of lost epidermis occurs through a process of epithelial migration from the edges of the wound and from any epithelial remnants left in the dermis. In most cases of nipple abrasion, the tissue that is lost is the superficial layer of the epidermis, which is healed by the acceleration of the normal process of basal cell maturation. Blistering may have a protective function for the rapid multiplication of basal cells. The fluid from the blister is absorbed rapidly if left alone.

DRY WOUND HEALING

When a tissue wound heals with exposure to air, the wound is able to breathe during the healing process; and a barrier of fibrin in the form of a scab appears. This

Figure 2A–2

Healing a fissure of the skin.

Source: Hole, JW (1981). *Human Anatomy and Physiology* (2nd ed.), p. 127. Dubuque, IA: William C. Brown Company. Copyright © 1981 Times Mirror Higher Education Group, Inc. All rights reserved. Reprinted with permission.

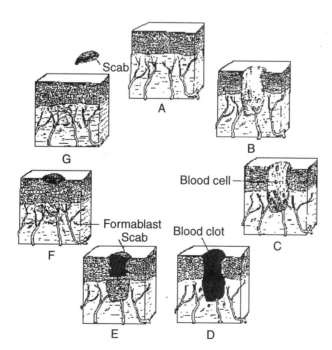

method of tissue healing requires covering the wound with a gauze bandage. When the scab falls off, it takes the newly formed tissue beneath it with it.

MOIST WOUND HEALING

Moist wound healing is presently thought of as an effective method of treating tissue wounds by many areas of the medical community. In moist wound healing, the wound heals under an occlusive or semi-occlusive medium. The wound is covered to prevent air exposure, and a medium that is permeable to water vapor and oxygen and is not penetrable to bacteria is applied. This method of wound healing retains internal moisture. Studies have shown rates of wound healing twice as fast in a moist environment as those allowed to heal in the drying air (Alper, 1983).

In cases of nipple abrasions or fissures, the tissue that is lost is the superficial layer of the epidermis, which is healed by the acceleration of the normal process of basal cell maturation. Scab formation, which occurs with dry wound healing, may present an impediment to the migration of epidermal cells across the surface of the wound. The retaining of internal moisture is believed to assist in the closure and healing of a fissure without the formation of a scab. Figures 2A–3 and 2A–4 show the normal migration of epithelial cells across the surface of the wound during the process of regeneration.

Internal moisture, which is desired in moist wound healing, is not to be confused with surface wetness, which is not desirable. Surface wetness, which may be present on the nipple immediately after nursing, contributes to nipple tenderness and damage if allowed to remain on the nipple area. Many mothers use brief exposure to room air or very gentle, light patting of the nipple area to dry the surface wetness after a breastfeeding session. Use of a blowdryer as a quick drying method is now being discouraged by many professionals—the rapid and excessive drying that occurs could lead to further cracking and damage of the already dehydrated tissues (Crase, 1992; Sharp, 1992).

Fissuring of the nipple may occur as the result of improper sucking or positioning of the infant at breast or inadequate moisture content in the layer of skin called the stratum corneum (Sharp, 1992). While identifying and eliminating the etiology of

Figure 2A–3
The process of regeneration.

Source: Courtesy of Lansinoh Laboratories. Reprinted with permission.

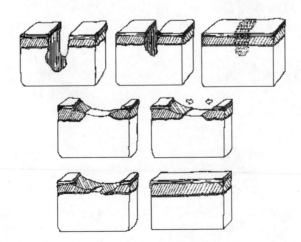

Figure 2A–4

Migration of epithelial cells during wound healing.

Source: Courtesy of Lansinoh Laboratories. Reprinted with permission.

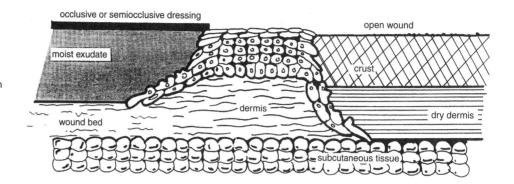

the nipple soreness/trauma remains a high priority, assisting the mother towards relief through treatment measures should also be important in order to avoid the possibility of premature weaning because of a worsening condition and pain.

To promote and complete the healing process while identifying and correcting the cause of the trauma, sufficient moisture should be reinstituted. This can be accomplished by the application of an appropriate medium, or "second skin," that meets the high standards of being suitable and safe for the breastfeeding mother's breasts and her breastfeeding infant. According to dermatologist Donald A. Sharp, MD (1992), "the application of an appropriate topical ointment, such as USP modified anhydrous lanolin, would be a dermatologist's first recommendation." A medical grade of anhydrous lanolin is one such appropriate medium for the breastfeeding mother. It does not inhibit air flow, but does suppress the evaporation of internal moisture while providing relief to the dry or cracked area (Crase, 1992; Sharp, 1992). Anhydrous lanolin is safe for the nursing mother and infant. The following list is representative of some of the factors that affect the repair process:

- Youth
- Adequate blood supply to affected area to bring oxygen to affected area and remove waste and debris from inflammatory process
- Good general health
- Adequate nutrient intake, especially protein and vitamin C which favor healing
- Minimal or moderate tissue destruction rather than extensive destruction
- An intact underlying framework upon which new tissues can be reconstructed
- The presence of tissues that are capable of regeneration

Nutrition and Wound Healing

Nutrition and wound healing is another area that must be considered. Evidence suggests that malnutrition has a significant effect on wound healing (Hadley & Fitzsimmons, 1990). Nutritional inadequacies may perplex the reparative mechanism in the process of healing (Hadley & Fitzsimmons, 1990; Levenson & Seifter, 1977). Inadequate nutritional intake and alterations in nutrient requirements or utilization, or both, may contribute to slowed wound healing, depressed immune function, and decreased resistance to infection (Hadley & Fitzsimmons, 1990; Levenson & Seifter, 1977; Reilly & Gerhardt, 1985). Wound healing and wound infection are areas that are integrated in that the metabolic and nutritional components influencing one of the areas will also play a role in influencing the other as well.

For wound healing to take place, sufficient nutritional stores and intake of protein, carbohydrates, fats, vitamins, and minerals are required. The following is a brief summary of the various nutritional factors and their roles in the wound-healing process.

B-Complex Vitamins—The B vitamins (riboflavin, thiamine, niacin, pyroxidine, and B_{12}) serve as cofactors in enzyme systems that affect the metabolism of protein, carbohydrate, and fat (Hadley & Fitzsimmons, 1990).

Carbohydrates—The body's preferred substrate for wound repair is glucose. Glucose serves as an energy source for leukocytes that engage in anti-inflammatory and phagocytic processes before fibroplasia (Ruberg, 1987).

Fats—The wound-healing function of fatty acids is not clear; however, it is known that fatty acids are needed for cell membranes and that fatty acids are anti-viral. Deficiencies in this area may impair the process of wound healing (Hadley & Fitzsimmons, 1990).

Minerals—The physiologic processes involved in wound healing require sufficient amounts of the electrolytes and macrominerals (sodium, potassium, chloride, phosphorus, magnesium) and the trace elements (iron, copper, manganese, and zinc). The macrominerals are integrated in functions that are essential for collagen formation, resistance to infection, and repair of damaged tissue. The trace minerals act as cofactors in enzyme systems that are also required for the wound-healing process (Hadley & Fitzsimmons, 1990; Levenson & Seifter, 1977; Ruberg, 1987).

Protein—Normal protein metabolism and nutrition are essential for wound healing. Cells synthesize and degrade their constituent proteins. Adequate proteins and amino acids are essential for the protein-synthesis and cell-multiplication processes of the healing wound. Clients/patients who are deficit in protein are at an increased risk for developing wound infections (Hadley & Fitzsimmons, 1990).

Vitamin A—Vitamin A fosters the wound-healing process by suppressing particular bacterial and fungal infections. It may also aid by counteracting the inhibitory effects of systemic steroid administration. A deficiency may impair epithelialization and closure of the open wound, healing of incisions of the skin, and the formation of reparative granulation tissues (Hadley & Fitzsimmons, 1990).

Vitamin C—Vitamin C (ascorbic acid) is essential for the hydroxylation of proline and lysine, a process that establishes the structure and function of the collagen molecule (Heughan, Grislis, & Hunt, 1974). A deficiency in ascorbic acid impairs the function of fibroblasts. Fibroblasts are responsible for the synthesis of collagen (Hadley & Fitzsimmons, 1990).

Vitamin K—Vitamin K is essential and required for the hepatic synthesis of clotting factors. Deficiencies in Vitamin K can cause defects in coagulation, which may lead to bleeding and hematoma formation (Hadley & Fitzsimmons, 1990).

Studies have repeatedly shown that nutritional deficiencies can impair the reparative process, thus impacting tissue healing. The tissue damage, as well as the person's nutritional status, is of high concern and should continually be considered in the overall care plan of the client (see Table 2A–1).

POST-TEST

For questions 1 to 6, choose the best answer:

1. _____ has bacteriostatic and fungicidal properties.
   A. Sebum
   B. Keratin
   C. Colostrum
   D. The sebaceous gland

2. The _____ has respiratory, excretory, and protection functions.
   A. keratin layer
   B. skin
   C. sebaceous gland
   D. areolar tissue

3. The blood vessels that nourish all the skin are located in the
   A. epidermis.
   B. dermis.
   C. keratin layer.
   D. None of the above.

4. _____ is a layer of protein accumulated on the epidermis layer of the skin.
   A. Sebum
   B. Galactorrhea
   C. Lactoprotein
   D. Keratin

5. The _____ is consistently sloughed off and replaced with a new layer, which enables the body to clean itself of adherent microorganisms.
   A. epidermis
   B. dermis
   C. keratin
   D. sebum

6. After _____ hardens and dries, a tough protective covering forms that prevents the escape of water from underlying tissues and the entry of various microorganisms.
   A. lactoprotein
   B. keratin
   C. sebaceous secreti
   D. epidermis

For questions 7 to 11, choose the best answer from the following key:

   A. Epidermis   **D. Sebaceous gland**
   B. Dermis   **E. Keratin**
   C. Sebum

7. _____ is composed of fibrous connective tissue.

8. _____ is composed of stratified squamous epithelium.

9. _____ helps protect the nipple and areola during sucking and also maintains an acid pH on the areola.

10. _____ is the tissue layer that is most often lost in nipple abrasions.

11. _____ protects underlying tissues against water loss and damage.

For questions 12 to 20, choose the best answer from the following key:
   A. True   B. False

12. The keratin layer is located on the skin's surface and is sloughed off to help eliminate microscopic metabolic waste.

13. Epidermal cells undergo keratinization as they are pushed toward the surface.

14. The epidermis accumulates a protein called sebum.

15. Nerve tissue is distributed throughout the dermis layer.

16. The areola contains sebaceous glands, which hypertrophy and form papillae during pregnancy.

17. Keratin is secreted by sebaceous glands.

18. The process of epithelialization is facilitated in moist dressed wounds, as compared with dry open wounds.

19. Studies have shown rates of wound healing that are twice as fast in a moist environment as those allowed to heal in the drying air.

20. Surface wetness is desirable in moist wound healing.

SECTION B

Nipple Soreness

Jan B. Simpson, RN, BSN, IBCLC

LEARNING OBJECTIVES

At the completion of this section, the learner will be able to do the following:

1. Discuss prenatal preparation of the nipples.
2. Identify and discuss possible causes of sore nipples and offer suggestions for prevention and management.
3. Assess the infant at breast, recognize possible problem areas, and assist the mother to correct them without undermining her confidence in her ability to nourish her infant.

OUTLINE

I. Introduction

II. Nipple Soreness Related to Positioning

    A. Causative factors

    B. Management suggestions

III. Nipple Soreness Related to Engorgement

    A. Causative factors

    B. Management suggestions

IV. Nipple Soreness Related to Early Introduction of Artificial Teats

    A. Causative factors

    B. Management suggestions

V. Nipple Soreness Related to Improper Removal of Infant from the Breast

    A. Causative factors

    B. Management suggestions

VI. Nipple Soreness Related to the Use of Creams and Ointments

    A. Causative factors

    B. Management suggestions

VII. Nipple Soreness Related to Bras and Bra Pads

    A. Causative factors

    B. Management suggestions

VIII. Nipple Soreness Related to Improper Positioning of Infant's Tongue

    A. Causative factors

    B. Management suggestions

IX. Nipple Soreness Related to Curling of Infant's Lip(s)

    A. Causative factors

    B. Management suggestions

X. Nipple Soreness Related to Candidiasis of the Nipple and Areolar Tissue

    A. Causative factors

    B. Management suggestions

XI. Nipple Soreness Related to Teething

    A. Causative factors

    B. Management suggestions

XII. Nipple Soreness Related to Improper Use of Breast Pumps

    A. Causative factors

    B. Management suggestions

XIII. Nipple Soreness Related to Unnecessary Cleaning of the Nipples

    A. Causative factors

    B. Management suggestions

PRE-TEST

For questions 1 to 11, choose the best answer.

1. A possible causative factor associated with nipple soreness is

    A. infant sucking on the breast with flanged lips.
    B. secretion of sebum by Montgomery's tubercles.
    C. improper positioning of the infant at breast.
    D. exposing the nipples to room air.

2. What prenatal preparation of the nipples is recommended for new mothers?

    A. Buffing nipples with towels
    B. Rolling nipples several times a day
    C. Exposure of nipple and areola area to air and indirect sunlight
    D. All of the above.

3. You would not recommend expressing breastmilk and air drying the nipples following a breastfeeding session

    A. when the tip of the nipple is sore.
    B. when a candida infection is present.
    C. when there is a nipple abrasion.
    D. when mastitis has been diagnosed.

4. Which best explains how the secretions of Montgomery's tubercles and the structure of the skin aid in maintaining skin integrity?

    A. The dermis layer is consistently sloughing, which rids the skin of microbes.
    B. Montgomery's tubercles secrete amino acids, which lowers the skin's pH and kills microbes.
    C. Sebum is an oily substance that has antimicrobial properties and, combined with the sloughing of the keratin layer, keeps the tissue healthy.
    D. Both B and C.

5. How might the early introduction of an artificial teat possibly cause problems for a mother wanting to breastfeed?

    A. It may cause nipple confusion in the infant.
    B. It will not cause a problem if introduction of an artificial teat is delayed until the infant is four days old.
    C. The infant uses a different action of the mouth, tongue, and mandible at the breast and bottle.
    D. Both A and C.
    E. Both B and C.

6. An appropriate way of removing the infant from the breast is

    A. inserting a clean finger into the infant's mouth and breaking the suction.
    B. pulling the infant off of the breast when the mother has finished breastfeeding.
    C. infant removes himself or herself from the breast when satisfied.
    D. Both A and C.

7. One recommendation that may be given when the mother is choosing a nursing bra:

    A. Wear a 100% cotton bra without underwire support or mid-cup seams
    B. Wear a 100% cotton bra with underwire support; no mid-cup seam
    C. Wear a bra that has a synthetic liner insert to help prevent leakage
    D. Both A and C.

8. Which best explains what to do if the nursing bra or bra pad is stuck to the nipple area by dried-on secretions?
   A. Apply dry heat using the low, warm setting of a blow dryer.
   B. Wet the bra and/or pad to remove it.
   C. Pour alcohol on the bra and/or pad. This will make removal easier and clean the nipple at the same time.
   D. Pull the bra or pad off quickly.

9. Suggestions for preventing nipple soreness caused by use of a breast pump include
   A. Center the nipple in the collection cup (flange) of the breast pump to avoid undue friction.
   B. Always begin pumping on the highest suction strength available, decreasing the strength slowly to a tolerable level.
   C. When using a breast pump that has a continuous negative pressure, hold the suction for one minute before releasing in order to obtain the highest milk yield.
   D. Both A and C.

10. Signs and symptoms of a candida infection of the nipple include
    A. mother complains of burning and stinging pains radiating up the breast during or between breastfeedings.
    B. sudden onset of painful nipples that do not respond to corrective treatment measures.
    C. nipples appear pink to red in color, with possible flaking, itching, or burning.
    D. All of the above.

11. Management suggestions for breastfeeding mothers with a candida infection include
    A. applying expressed breastmilk to the nipple.
    B. treating the infant's mouth with an antifungal medication.
    C. treating the mother's nipple and areola and the infant's mouth with an antifungal medication.
    D. applying anhydrous lanolin to the nipple and areola.

For questions 12 to 20, choose the best answer from the following key:

A. True   B. False

12. When assessing the infant at breast, the infant's mouth should be opened widely and his lips flanged outward.

13. The tongue should be extended over the lower alveolar ridge while the infant is actively nursing.

14. Smacking sounds are excellent indicators that the infant is obtaining milk from the breast.

15. When the infant is sucking at the breast, his cheeks should have an obvious dimpling, or drawing in, to indicate a good suction.

16. Creams or ointments used on the breast should contain alcohol.

17. Creams or ointments used on the breast should contain antibiotics.

18. If the breasts become engorged, the mother's nipples tend to protract, making latch-on easier in some cases.

19. Application of ice to engorged breasts following a breastfeeding session is no longer recommended because it has been found to inhibit the milk-ejection reflex and milk flow at the next feeding.

20. The removal of milk from the mother's breast occurs by the peristaltic-like movement of the infant's tongue and the opening and closing action of the infant's mandible.

Introduction

Sore nipples are one of the most common problems that women associate with a negative breastfeeding experience. Many women report nipple soreness in the first week postpartum, with improvement thereafter. Sore nipples do not have to occur; but if they become sore and the discomfort lasts throughout the entire feeding, something is wrong. If the breastfeeding mother complains of pain, look for the etiology and work with the mother to help correct the problem and alleviate the pain before further complications occur. Do not limit the infant's time at the breast under the misconception that this will prevent or limit nipple soreness. Limiting time does not prevent nipple soreness; it only delays it (Whitley, 1974). It may also end the breastfeeding session prematurely, before the milk-ejection reflex has occurred, or prevent the infant from obtaining the hindmilk (Riordan & Auerbach, 1993). If managed inappropriately, sore nipples can lead to further complications, including: cracked nipples, bleeding nipples, blistered nipples, infections, or even untimely weaning of the infant from the breast (Neville & Neifert, 1983).

Prenatal preparation of the nipples by mothers who plan to breastfeed not only does little to prevent nipple soreness (Walker & Driscoll, 1989) but may be the beginning of nipple problems. Buffing the nipples with towels or other abrasive objects or rough manipulation of the nipples in order to prepare them for the infant's suck is not recommended. Nipple damage can occur by the continued removal of the skin's keratin layer. Continuous removal of the natural oils of the nipple and areola may predispose the skin to irritation. The Montgomery tubercles of the areola secrete a sebaceous substance that cleans and lubricates the areola and nipple. This should not be removed. Bathing as usual and avoiding soap or any drying substance on the nipple area is advised. Uterine contractions may occur by the rough handling, rolling, and pulling of the nipples. Prenatal clients should be encouraged to prepare their minds for breastfeeding instead of their nipples. Exposure of the breasts to air and mild sunlight, or the light friction received from going braless or wearing a nursing bra with the flaps down for short periods of time, is more than adequate preparation. Lovemaking with gentle involvement of the breasts is typically harmless in most cases and is an effectual preparation (Hewat & Ellis, 1987; Lawrence, 1989).

The most common etiology of sore nipples in the first few days after giving birth is usually related to improper positioning or latching-on of the infant to the breast (Lawrence, 1989). Possible causative factors may include one or more of the following: improper positioning, improper latch-on, engorgement, early introduction of artificial teats, nipple shields, improper removal of infant from breast, sensitivity to breast creams or ointments, plastic liners in breast or breast pads, improper positioning of infant's tongue while nursing, infant's lip or lips curled under while nursing (not flanged), candidiasis (thrush), teething, improper use of or unrelieved negative pressure from breast pumps, unnecessary cleaning of nipples, and ankyloglossia (Hazelbaker, 1993; Lawrence, 1989; Neville & Neifert, 1983; Riordan & Auerbach, 1993; Walker & Driscoll, 1989). Table 2B–1 summarizes most of the possible causes of nipple soreness.

Table 2B–1   Possible Causative Factors of Sore Nipples

- Improper positioning of infant at the breast
- Improper latch-on
- Engorgement
- Early introduction of artificial teats
- Nipple shields
- Improper removal of infant from breast
- Breast creams and ointments
- Plastic liners in bras or bra pads
- Improper positioning of infant's tongue while nursing
- Improper use of breast pumps
- Unrelieved negative pressure
- Unnecessary cleaning of the nipples
- Ankyloglossia
- Candidiasis
- Teething
- Infant's lip or lips are curled under or pursed while nursing (not flanged)

Nipple Soreness Related to Positioning

CAUSATIVE FACTORS

Poor positioning of the infant at the breast can cause nipple soreness. However, the breastfeeding mother who is knowledgeable and accomplishes correct positioning and latching-on of the infant may have little, if any, initial nipple tenderness. While in the hospital, where breastfeeding assistance can be obtained easily, the breastfeeding mother should be taught proper positioning and effective latch-on techniques. Guidelines for evaluating positioning are provided in Chapter 1 of this module.

The health-care professionals assisting the mother and infant with breastfeeding should evaluate the infant at the breast and assess the need for intervention teaching. Several tools for assessing the infant at the breast have appeared in the literature. These are the Systematic Assessment of the Infant at Breast (SAIB) (Shrago & Bocar, 1990), the Mother–Baby Assessment for Breastfeeding (MBA) (Mulford, 1992), the Vancouver Breastfeeding Centre tool (Ellis, Livingstone, & Hewat, 1993), the Infant Breastfeeding Assessment Tool (Matthews, 1988), the B-R-E-A-S-T observation form (Armstrong, 1990), and the LATCH tool (Jensen, Wallace, & Kelsay, 1994). See Chapter 1 in this module for a description of these tools.

MANAGEMENT SUGGESTIONS FOR NIPPLE SORENESS RELATED TO POSITIONING

1. Evaluate the infant at breast while teaching the client positioning and latch-on techniques (see Figure 2B–1).
2. When evaluating the infant at breast, include an assessment of the steps from one of the assessment tools. During the production and secretion of colostrum by the mother, it is not always possible to hear swallowing.
3. Inspect the mother's breasts. Oftentimes the area of trauma may assist you in determining the etiology of soreness.

   a. If cracking of the nipple tissue is noted on the underside, it is possible that the etiology is too much of the top areola or too little of the bottom is being taken into the infant's mouth (Riordan & Auerbach, 1993). It may also be related to the infant keeping his lower lip curled under instead of being properly flanged outward (Maher, 1988; Walker & Driscoll, 1989)—see Figure 2B–2.

   b. If complaints of soreness or trauma are occurring in the area of 10 to 12 o'clock and 4 to 6 o'clock positions on the right breast, or 12 to 2 o'clock and 6 to 8 o'clock on the left breast, it is possibly due to the infant sucking too low on the breast or too close to the nipple tip (Riordan & Auerbach, 1993).

   c. Bruising that appears crescent-shaped and is located above or below the nipple base may be due to the infant not latching on to the nipple and areola far enough beyond the base of the nipple (Walker & Driscoll, 1989).

Figure 2B–1

Proper positioning of infant at breast using cradle-hold position.

Source: Renfrew, M, Fisher, C, Arms, S (1990). *Breastfeeding: Getting Breastfeeding Right for You*, pp. 80 and 85. Copyright © 1990 by Mary Renfrew, Chloe Fisher, and Suzanne Arms. Reprinted with permission of Celestial Arts, Berkeley, CA.

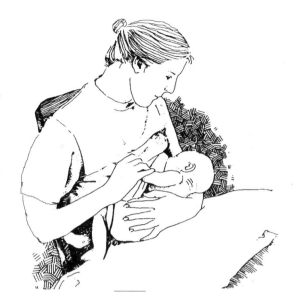

Figure 2B–2

Infant latched on to breast showing properly flanged lips.

Source: Renfrew, M, Fisher, C, Arms, S (1990). *Breastfeeding: Getting Breastfeeding Right for You*, pp. 80 and 85. Copyright © 1990 by Mary Renfrew, Chloe Fisher, and Suzanne Arms. Reprinted with permission of Celestial Arts, Berkeley, CA.

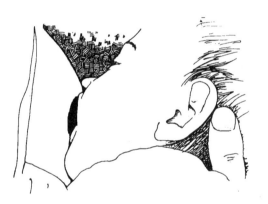

    d. When the infant is removed from the breast and the nipple tip appears white or blanched, the infant may be pinching the nipple between the upper and lower alveolar ridges or compressing the nipple excessively when swallowing (Walker & Driscoll, 1989).

    e. A red stripe located diagonally in the midline of the nipple or a visible blanched crease in the nipple may be due to the infant's tongue retracting behind the lower alveolar ridge (Walker & Driscoll, 1989).

4. Encourage the client/patient to change nursing positions frequently in order to change pressure areas on the breast and empty as many lactiferous sinuses as possible.

Nipple Soreness Related to Engorgement

CAUSATIVE FACTORS

If the breasts become engorged, the mother's nipples tend to become flattened and the areola hard. This makes it extremely difficult for the infant to latch on to the breasts properly. The firmness of the areola causes the infant to grasp the end of the nipple, which leads to nipple soreness and probably exacerbation of the engorgement because of inadequate emptying of milk from the breast. Management of engorgement is further explained in Section C of this chapter.

MANAGEMENT SUGGESTIONS FOR NIPPLE SORENESS RELATED TO ENGORGEMENT

1. Prior to breastfeeding, use warm, moist compresses and gentle breast massage to stimulate a milk-ejection reflex and help the milk flow. Some mothers may prefer a warm shower, gently massaging while in the shower, or leaning over and placing the breasts in a basin of warm water (Lauwers & Woessner, 1989; Lawrence, 1989; Neville & Neifert, 1983). Heat is a vasodilator and should only be used to elicit a milk-ejection reflex in a breast with physiologic engorgement. In physiologic engorgement, heat and manual expression can soften the areola adequately for infant latch-on. In cases of pathologic engorgement, heat will make the situation worsen. Physiologic and pathologic engorgement are discussed in the next section of this chapter. Ice or cabbage leaves will reduce swelling that accompanies pathologic engorgement and, when accompanied by gentle breast massage and areolar compression, the nipple can be softened for achieving latch-on.

2. If the infant is having difficulty latching on due to engorgement of the areola, gently, manually express just enough milk to soften the areola so the infant may achieve proper latch-on (Lauwers & Woessner, 1990; Lawrence, 1989).

3. Suggest that the mother try various nursing positions to find one that may assist her in latching the infant on to the breast properly. Many mothers find the football or clutch hold especially helpful when nursing on an engorged breast.

4. Application of ice following a breastfeeding session may help relieve swelling and promote comfort.

Nipple Soreness Related to Early Introduction of Artificial Teats

CAUSATIVE FACTORS

Sucking from a rubber teat on a bottle requires different mouth and tongue performance than sucking on the mother's breast (Neville and Neifert, 1983). When an infant is given a rubber teat on a bottle, the mouth must only open a small amount, with the lips closed around the small rubber teat. The tongue is thrust forward, but peristalsis of the tongue does not occur due to the rapid flow of liquid from the artificial teat opening (Ardran, Kemp, & Lind, 1958; Lawrence, 1989). Little if any action is required by the mandible.

When sucking from the mother's breast, the infant's mouth is opened wide and his lips are flanged outward, forming a seal around the large portion of breast that has been taken in. The tongue is extended beyond the lower alveolar ridge, forming a trough and cupping under the breast. The tongue will remain in place here throughout the breastfeeding (Weber, Woolridge, & Baum, 1986). The removal of milk from the mother's breast occurs by the peristaltic-like movement of the infant's tongue and the opening and closing action of the mandible. The closing action of the mandible expresses breastmilk from the lactiferous sinuses of the breast to the back of the infant's oral cavity. As the opening action of the mandible occurs, the lactiferous sinuses are refilled (Woolridge, 1986).

Due to the different actions required when sucking from a bottle or sucking on the breast, nipple confusion may occur from even a few supplemental or complementary bottles given. Some young infants are unable to make the change back and forth from breast to bottle. In nipple confusion, the infant's tongue is not properly placed over the lower alveolar ridge, cupping the breast, thus causing sore nipples. A drawing in or dimpling of the cheeks may be observed and a clicking sound may be heard, indicating a dysfunctional suck at the breast.

MANAGEMENT SUGGESTIONS FOR NIPPLE SORENESS RELATED TO EARLY INTRODUCTION OF ARTIFICIAL TEATS

1. Breastfeeding mothers should be encouraged to breastfeed exclusively, without the introduction of rubber teats/bottles, for the first four to six weeks of life. This assists in establishing her milk supply and avoids possible nipple confusion for her infant.

2. If supplemental or complement feeds must be given, suggest feeding with a cup, spoon, dropper, finger, or using a nursing supplemental system. See Chapter 3 in this module for a discussion on the use of alternative feeding methods.

Nipple Soreness Related to Improper Removal of Infant from the Breast

CAUSATIVE FACTORS

Routine removal of the infant from the breast without releasing the suction can lead to nipple soreness and tissue breakdown, which may lead to further complications. The breastfeeding mother should be encouraged to nurse until the infant spontaneously removes himself or herself from the breast and appears to be satisfied (see Figure 2B–3) or, if removal is mother-initiated, by inserting a clean finger into the infant's mouth between the upper and lower alveolar ridges and releasing the suction.

MANAGEMENT SUGGESTIONS FOR NIPPLE SORENESS RELATED TO THE IMPROPER REMOVAL OF THE INFANT FROM THE BREAST

1. Encourage the mother to allow the infant to end the feeding at each breast.
2. When the feeding must be stopped by the mother, instruct her to break the suction first by sliding her finger between the upper and lower alveolar ridges in the infant's mouth.

Figure 2B–3

Ending the feeding.

Source: Renfrew, M, Fisher, C, Arms, S (1990). *Breastfeeding: Getting Breastfeeding Right for You*, p. 191. Copyright © 1990 by Mary Renfrew, Chloe Fisher, and Suzanne Arms. Reprinted with permission of Celestial Arts, Berkeley, CA.

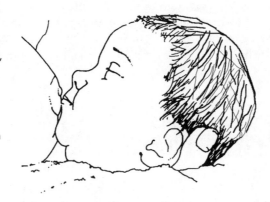

Nipple Soreness Related to the Use of Creams and Ointments

CAUSATIVE FACTORS

Occasionally a cream or ointment may cause a dermatitis of the skin of the mother's nipple and areola. Through the years, mothers who are allergic to wool or have a strong familial history of allergies have been cautioned against the use of lanolin. If an irritation appears while using any type of nipple cream or ointment, discontinue its use immediately. Creams and ointments have also been known to possibly change the taste of the nipple. Using them may initiate fussiness in the infant or a complete refusal of the breast.

The free-lanolin alcohol found naturally in lanolins has been identified as the allergic component in lanolin. The higher the free-lanolin alcohol content is, the greater the incidence of allergic responses (Clark, 1993; Clark et al., 1977). Clinical trials have indicated that at a level of 6.5% free-lanolin alcohol, 41% of a lanolin-sensitive population continue to experience an allergic response (Clark, 1975). Even with the free-lanolin alcohol decreased to 3% and 2.2%, allergic responses were documented. Only when the level of free-lanolin alcohol was reduced to 1.5% and the detergent content was insignificant were researchers unable to detect any allergic response among those who were considered to be sensitive to lanolin (Clark et al., 1977).

New standards governing the requirements and limitations for lanolin products became effective on May 15, 1992. The U.S. Pharmacopeial Convention (USP) set "the limitation of pesticide residues for modified lanolin at not more than 1 ppm of any individual pesticide and not more than a total of 3 ppm of all pesticide residues. Additionally, the monograph limits the content of free lanolin alcohols to not more than 6%" (U.S. Pharmacopeial Convention, 1992).

Breast creams and ointments are once again at the center of controversy—recent clinical research has suggested that the use of modified lanolin is associated with accelerated healing of severely dry and cracked nipples (Huggins & Billion, 1993; Spangler & Hildebrandt, 1993). Table 2B–2 lists some important things to consider when selecting an appropriate topical for the breast.

A medical-grade, modified version of lanolin called Lansinoh (see Figure 2B–4) is now receiving attention. Lansinoh, manufactured by Lansinoh Laboratories (Western Springs, IL), is an ultrapure, modified lanolin that is registered with the U.S. Food and Drug Administration (FDA) as an over-the-counter (OTC) drug. Lansinoh Laboratories guarantees that the product never exceeds the limit of 1.5% free-lanolin alcohols, which makes it truly hypoallergenic according to the results of Clark et al. (1977), never contains in excess of 0.05 detergent residue, and contains less than 1 ppm or ten thousandths of 1% total combined pesticide residue (Sue Huml, Lansinoh Laboratories, personal communication, 1995). These criteria exceed the standards set by the USP. La Leche League International (LLLI) officially endorsed Lansinoh as the product of choice to relieve pain and aid healing, thus enabling the mother with sore nipples to continue to breastfeed (LLLI, 1993).

Medela, Inc., offers Purelan® 100 (Medela, 1993). Purelan 100 is reported by Medela (manufacturer) to contain less than 3% free-lanolin alcohols and less than

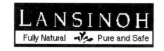

Figure 2B–4

An over-the-counter form of lanolin.

Table 2B-2   Selecting an Appropriate Topical for the Breast

The answer should be "no" to the following questions:

1. Does the cream/ointment need to be removed from the breast prior to nursing?
2. Could the cream/ointment clog pores or block milk ducts?
3. Does the cream/ointment contain multi-ingredients?
4. Does the cream/ointment alter the pH balance of the skin?
5. Does the cream/ointment make the nipple feel slippery?

The answer should be "yes" to the following questions:

1. Is the cream/ointment safe for the infant to ingest?
2. Is the cream/ointment hypoallergenic?
3. Is the cream/ointment bacteriostatic?
4. Is the cream/ointment completely pure and safe?

Source: Huml, SC (June 1993). Applying Moist Wound Healing Principles to the Healing of Fissured Nipples in the Breastfeeding Mother. From lecture outline for IBCLC, June 1993. Reprinted with permission.

3 ppm of all combined pesticides. These criteria also meet the standards set by the USP. But the free-lanolin alcohols in Purelan 100 may exceed the level of 1.5% found to be safe for women who had experienced sensitivity to lanolin (Clark et al., 1977).

The use of the mother's own expressed colostrum or hindmilk following a breastfeeding session should continue to be strongly encouraged as the number one cream to use on the nipple area. Breastmilk contains antibacterial and antiviral properties, as well as other immune bodies. Reports have documented the healing components of breastmilk when applied to sore nipples (Lawrence, 1989). If the mother prefers to use a commercial cream to lubricate the skin of the nipple area, she should be cautioned about the types of creams and ointments to avoid, in addition to proper application techniques.

MANAGEMENT SUGGESTIONS FOR NIPPLE SORENESS RELATED TO USE OF CREAMS AND OINTMENTS

1. Teach the breastfeeding mother about the sebaceous glands (called Montgomery's tubercles), which secrete the body's own natural cream (called sebum). Sebum has bacteriostatic and fungicidal properties (Hole, 1981).

2. Strongly encourage the breastfeeding mother to express a few drops of her colostrum or hindmilk at the end of a breastfeeding session and gently rub it into the skin, unless the mother has candidiasis on her nipples.

3. Stress the importance of air drying or gently patting the nipples prior to applying a recommended commercial cream or ointment in order to avoid sealing in surface moisture and delaying healing.

4. Make the nursing mother who chooses to use an artificial cream aware that some artificial breast creams and ointments have been noted to change the taste of the nipple and may cause fussiness or breast refusal in the infant.

5. Instruct the mother to immediately discontinue use of any cream or ointment if irritation occurs.

Nipple Soreness Related
to Bras and Bra Pads

CAUSATIVE FACTORS

Discourage the breastfeeding mother from wearing bras or nursing pads that have any type of plastic liner or synthetic fiber, because they tend to hold in moisture and promote nipple soreness. If leaking occurs and the bra or nursing pad becomes stuck to the nipple, instruct the mother to moisten it with water before removing it in order to prevent further nipple damage.

Another common source of sore nipples is continuous wearing of a bra that is too tight. Encourage the mother to purchase and wear a comfortable bra of the correct cup size, without an underwire. Many women with large breasts prefer underwire styles, and a proper fit is imperative to avoid undue pressure on the ducts in the lower areas of the breasts. Lactation consultants should learn how to properly fit a bra.

An additional culprit related to sore nipples is a bra that has a rough seam located midline in the bra cup. Encourage the use of a seamless bra, if possible.

MANAGEMENT SUGGESTIONS FOR NIPPLE
SORENESS RELATED TO BRAS
AND BRA PADS

1. Encourage use of bra pads without plastic liners. Many women prefer to use disposable bra pads. Plastic liners tend to hold in moisture and create an excellent environment for tender nipples and infection. Offer the suggestion of using a cut-up 100% cotton T-shirt or handkerchief for homemade reusable bra pads.

2. Encourage use of 100% cotton bras that do not have plastic liners, which tend to hold in moisture and create an excellent environment for tender nipples and infection.

3. Discourage the use of bras with underwires because they may compress areas of the breast, blocking lactiferous ducts and predisposing the breastfeeding mother to plugged ducts and mastitis. If a woman prefers an underwire style, appropriate fit is a must.

4. Instruct the mother to moisten the bra or nursing pad before removing it if it becomes stuck to the nipple area to avoid tissue injury.

Nipple Soreness Related to Improper Positioning of Infant's Tongue

CAUSATIVE FACTORS

Improper positioning of the infant's tongue while at the breast causes an inadequate suck; however, this can be corrected. This common cause of nipple soreness can also have an effect on the maternal milk production.

The infant's tongue should form a trough and be extended beyond the lower alveolar ridge. The breastfeeding mother, or caregiver assessing the feeding session, can visually assess the positioning of the tongue by gently pulling the lower lip down while the infant is sucking. Movement of the tongue over the lower alveolar ridge should be noted. If the tongue cannot be seen and the mother is feeling discomfort, hears a clicking or smacking sound, or sees dimpling of the infant's cheeks, suction should be broken, the infant removed from the breast, and latch-on begun again. The infant may have incorrect positioning of the tongue (see Figure 2B–5).

In some, but not all, cases a digital examination is indicated. In a digital exam, a clean finger is inserted into the infant's mouth with the finger pad side up. The infant's tongue should form a trough, cupping the examiner's finger. Sucking by the infant is usually begun as the pad of the finger touches the palate. This should never be done before the infant has been put to breast for the first time.

MANAGEMENT SUGGESTIONS FOR NIPPLE SORENESS RELATED TO IMPROPER POSITIONING OF INFANT'S TONGUE

1. Assess the infant at breast for proper tongue positioning. Teach the mother to do this also.

2. Instruct the breastfeeding mother on signs of an effective suck. See Chapter 1 in this module for more information on assessing the infant at the breast.

3. Refer to Section D in this chapter for causes and management of sucking difficulties.

Figure 2B–5

Incorrect positioning of the tongue unless the infant has ankyloglossia.

Source: Minchin, M (1985). *Breastfeeding Matters—What We Need to Know About Infant Feeding*, p. 88. Victoria, Australia: Alma Publications and George Allen and Unwin. Reprinted with permission.

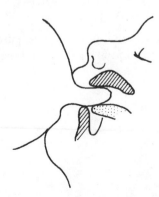

Nipple Soreness Related to Curling of Infant's Lip(s)

CAUSATIVE FACTORS

The infant's lips should appear flanged outward while nursing at the breast. If the mother notes that the breastfeeding infant's upper and/or lower lip is curled under, she should gently pull the lip out while the infant continues to suck. Curled-in lips can be a cause of sore nipples. If the breastfeeding mother complains of soreness on the underside of the nipple, the infant's bottom lip may be curled in, causing friction abrasion (Lawrence, 1989; Walker & Driscoll, 1989).

MANAGEMENT SUGGESTIONS FOR NIPPLE SORENESS RELATED TO CURLING OF INFANT'S LIP(S)

1. Assess the infant at breast for proper latch-on and lip positioning. Teach the breastfeeding mother self-assessment techniques.
2. Instruct the breastfeeding mother to gently pull out the infant's curled lips with her finger while breastfeeding if necessary to assist them to an outwardly flanged position.

Nipple Soreness Related to Candidiasis of the Nipple and Areolar Tissue

CAUSATIVE FACTORS

Candidiasis is an infection caused by a genus of yeast called *Candida*. An organism called *Candida albicans* is the most common etiologic agent, although involvement by other species is possible (Wei, 1988). *C. albicans* thrives on milk and warm, moist areas, such as the breastfeeding infant's mouth and perianal area and the nursing mother's nipples and vagina.

Candidiasis can occur at any time during the breastfeeding relationship and should be suspected if the mother complains of suddenly occurring painful nipples that do not respond to typical treatment measures. Other signs and symptoms of possible candidiasis involving the nipple area include pink or red nipples and areolae that have the appearance of flaking or peeling and complaints of nipple and areolar itching. The absence of signs and symptoms of a candida infection in the infant does not rule out candida infection of the mother. The infant may oftentimes appear to be asymptomatic. See Section C in this chapter for a more extensive discussion of candidiasis.

MANAGEMENT SUGGESTIONS FOR CANDIDIASIS OF THE NIPPLE AND AREOLAR TISSUE

1. Both mother and infant must be treated simultaneously if candidiasis occurs. If only one is treated, the infection will continue to be passed back and forth between mother and infant. If the infection continues to occur after treatments, possible treatment of the mother's partner should be considered.

2. The mother should contact her physician or public health nurse practitioner for prescription medication to treat the infant's mouth, her nipples, and possibly the infant's bottom or the mother's vagina. Treatments should be effective within 1 to 3 days for milder infections and 5 to 10 days for more severe infections. Simultaneous treatment should continue for the entire course of the medication, even if candidiasis appears to have disappeared.

3. The mother should expose her nipples to air and indirect sunlight during the day, when possible (Riordan, 1991). She should make an effort to keep the nipple area as dry as possible, changing bra pads and bras as necessary when they become moist. The mother should be advised to avoid applying creams or ointments.

4. The mother should sterilize all objects that come in contact with the infant's mouth (pacifiers/dummies, teething rings) or her breasts (bras, bra pads, breast shells).

Nipple Soreness Related to Teething

CAUSATIVE FACTORS

When an infant is teething and has a tooth about to erupt, he or she may have swelling and irritation of the gums. Teething may present a temporary obstacle in the breastfeeding relationship for some, because it may lead to biting as the infant discovers that chewing helps reduce teething discomfort.

Many breastfeeding mothers believe that once their infant begins teething, or the first tooth erupts, they must wean immediately. This is not true. If the infant begins to chew on the nipple because of swollen or sore gums, and the mother begins to complain of sore nipples, offer reassurance and encouragement that this is for a brief period and only temporary. Offer other suggestions of relief measures for the teething infant. She can rub the infant's gums or offer a cool teething ring or cool cloth to chew on. Encourage her to always check with her pediatric dentist or pediatrician before applying any type of numbing medication to the infant's gums because numbing of the tongue and the gag reflex could occur.

If the infant begins biting, this is a sign that he or she is no longer actively nursing. When an infant is actively nursing, the tongue is extended beyond the lower gum ridge, between the teeth and the breast, and the nipple is drawn far into the back of the infant's mouth. Some infants may begin to chew on the nipple at the end of a feeding or when playing. Encourage the mother to watch for signs that a feeding is over. Some infants begin to chew on the nipple when they fall asleep at the breast. Again, the feeding is over, and the infant should be removed from the breast.

Many infants never bite when breastfeeding, but there are those who do. Usually, the startled response of the mother discourages the infant from biting again. If the biting continues, other measures may be taken, such as stopping the feeding and offering the infant another object to chew.

MANAGEMENT SUGGESTIONS FOR NIPPLE SORENESS RELATED TO TEETHING

1. Encourage the breastfeeding mother to learn to recognize signs that her infant is nearing the end of a breastfeeding session. During teething, when the mother feels the infant's tongue retract back into the mouth, and it is no longer extended over the lower alveolar ridge, suction should be broken, and the infant should be removed from the breast.

2. Offer suggestions for comforting the teething infant, such as massaging the gums with a finger or cold washcloth, offering teething rings, etc., prior to breastfeeding, so breastfeeding sessions may be more comfortable for the baby.

3. Remind the breastfeeding mother that this is a temporary situation.

Nipple Soreness Related to Improper Use of Breast Pumps

CAUSATIVE FACTORS

There are many types of breast pumps available to the breastfeeding mother. If the pump is not used correctly, nipple damage can occur. The "bicycle horn" pump causes damage to the nipple because there is no way to regulate suction and because it cannot be adequately cleaned between pumping sessions (Lauwers & Woessner, 1990). Many of the battery- or AC adapter–controlled pumps have a continuous negative pressure, which can cause damaged nipples if the mother does not follow instructions carefully and relieve the suction. Cylinder-type pumps can also cause sore nipples because of the continuous negative pressure suction applied by the mother. When there is not an automatic release of suction by the pump, depending on the type pump being used, instruct the mother that continuous or lengthy negative pressure may damage her nipples.

The mother should always make sure the nipple is centered in the middle of the pump flange to avoid any undue friction. She should always begin pumping on the least suction strength available, gradually increasing the suction strength to a comfortable level during the pumping session.

See Chapter 3 in this module for a discussion of breast pumps.

MANAGEMENT SUGGESTIONS FOR NIPPLE SORENESS RELATED TO IMPROPER USE OF BREAST PUMPS

1. Encourage the use of a physiological pump, a pump with automatic suction release or automatic cycling, when possible.
2. When using a pump with continuous negative pressure, caution the mother to release suction frequently, as per instructions.
3. Avoid using a bicycle horn–style pump.
4. The nipple should be centered in the middle of the pump flange to avoid any undue rubbing against plastic pump parts.
5. Always start pumping on the least suction strength available, gradually increasing it throughout a feeding to a comfortable, productive strength.
6. Never remove the breast pump from the breast unless the suction is off.
7. Individual pump parts should not be shared between mothers to avoid passing microbes between them.

Nipple Soreness Related to Unnecessary Cleaning of the Nipples

CAUSATIVE FACTORS

The woman who plans to breastfeed or who is breastfeeding should avoid all soaps, alcohol, or any drying agents on the breasts. A daily shower, with plain water to the nipples, is more than adequate. It is not necessary to wash the breast or nipple area before each feeding session. The harshness of a washcloth will remove the keratin layer of skin, predisposing the nipples to soreness, as well as washing away the protective oils naturally produced by Montgomery's tubercles.

MANAGEMENT SUGGESTIONS FOR NIPPLE SORENESS RELATED TO UNNECESSARY CLEANING OF THE NIPPLES

1. Encourage the mother to wash her hands, not her nipples, each time before breastfeeding.

2. A daily shower, with plain water to the nipples, is all that is necessary to keep the nipples clean for breastfeeding.

3. Avoid soaps and any other drying agents, such as alcohol, to the nipple area. Soaps, alcohol, and tincture of Benzoin have been reported to cause tissue damage of the areola and nipple (Lawrence, 1989; Neifert & Seacat, 1986). Soap not only removes the natural oils of the skin, but it interferes with the natural acid–alkaline balance.

4. The breastfeeding mother should be instructed not to scrub her nipples. This action can remove and destroy the natural oils and could cause drying and cracking of the tissues.

5. No commercial artificial creams or ointments are indicated if the natural oils of the areola and nipple have not been removed.

POST-TEST

For questions 1 to 5, choose the best answer from the following key:

A. if responses 1, 2, and 3 are correct   C. if responses 2 and 4 are correct
B. if responses 1 and 3 are correct   D. if all responses are correct

1. Nipple soreness can be caused by
    1. the infant sucking at the breast with only one lip curled under.
    2. exposing the nipples to room air.
    3. the infant's head not in straight alignment with his body while nursing.
    4. secretion of sebum by Montgomery's tubercles.

2. _____ is recommended prenatally for mothers planning to breastfeed.
    1. Talking to her physician about breastfeeding
    2. Exposing the nipple and areola areas to air and indirect sunlight
    3. Attending breastfeeding support groups
    4. Buffing nipples with towels

3. Cracking of the tissue on the underneath side of the nipple and areola is
    1. caused by too little of the bottom part of the areola being taken into the infant's mouth.
    2. caused by too much of the top part of the areola being taken into the infant's mouth.
    3. caused by the infant keeping his lower lip curled under instead of being properly flanged outward.
    4. caused by the infant keeping his upper lip curled under instead of being properly flanged outward.

4. A mother complains of nipple trauma on her right breast occurring in the 12 o'clock position. This is
    1. caused by the infant sucking too low on the breast area.
    2. caused by candida infection.
    3. caused by the infant sucking too close to the nipple tip.
    4. normal and will heal in time.

5. Bruising that appears crescent-shaped and is located above or below the nipple base may be due to
    A. the infant not latching on to the nipple and areola far enough.
    B. the asymmetrical buildup of the keratin layer of skin.
    C. the infant not taking the nipple and areola in his mouth appropriately.
    D. a candida infection.

For questions 6 to 9, choose the best answer.

6. Which of the following best describes nipple confusion?
    A. Different action of the mouth, tongue, and mandible that occurs when sucking from the breast and the bottle
    B. Does not occur if early introduction of artificial teats is delayed until the infant is four days old
    C. Different tongue action required as the infant goes from breast to bottle
    D. An old wives' tale

7. When the infant is removed from the breast and the nipple tip appears white or blanched, it may be due to
   A. a candida infection.
   B. the infant compressing the nipple excessively when swallowing.
   C. the infant pinching the nipple between the upper and lower alveolar ridges.
   D. Both B and C.
   E. Both A and C.

8. A red stripe located diagonally in the midline of the nipple or a visibly blanched crease may be due to
   A. a candida infection.
   B. galactorrhea.
   C. the infant's tongue retracting behind the lower alveolar ridge.
   D. Both A and C.
   E. Both B and C.

9. A mother complains that areas of her nipple are a deep red/purple color. You suspect that this may be due to
   A. an abscess.
   B. mastitis.
   C. incorrect attachment of the infant to the breast.
   D. None of the above.

For questions 10 to 15, choose the best answer from the following key:
   A. True
   B. False

10. A nursing bra with mid-cup seams may be a possible cause of sore nipples.

11. To remove a bra or bra pad that is stuck to the nipple area, pour alcohol on the nipple area to loosen the materials and clean the nipple simultaneously.

12. Gloves should be worn by the mother with a candida infection when breastfeeding her infant to help prevent contamination of the infant.

13. Candida infection may be suspected if the mother complains of burning and stinging pains radiating up the breast during or between feedings.

14. The client should be encouraged to change nursing positions frequently in order to change pressure areas on the breast and empty as many lactiferous sinuses as possible.

15. Montgomery's tubercles (glands) secrete a substance called keratin, which has bacteriostatic and fungicidal properties.

For questions 16 to 20, choose the best answer from the following key:
   A. appropriate
   B. inappropriate

16. Removing the sebum from the nipples prior to breastfeeding is _____.

17. Applying a cream or ointment on the breast that has instructions to remove prior to breastfeeding or not for ingestion is _____.

18. Expressing a few drops of colostrum or hindmilk at the end of a feeding, gently patting it on the nipple area, and allowing it to dry is _____.

19. Air drying or gently patting the nipple area following a breastfeeding session to remove surface wetness prior to applying a recommended artificial cream or ointment is _____.

20. Applying tincture of Benzoin to sore nipples is _____.

SECTION C

Breast-Related Problems

Jan B. Simpson, RN, BSN, IBCLC

LEARNING OBJECTIVES

At the completion of this section, the learner will be able to do the following:

1. Recognize signs and symptoms of candidiasis and advise the breastfeeding mother of an appropriate plan of care.

2. Discuss the effects of herpes simplex virus on the breastfeeding relationship, offering recommendations for the lactating mother during a period of outbreak.

3. Identify various classifications of nipple function, offering ways to help manage ungraspable nipples for breastfeeding success.

4. Identify possible causes of nipple discharge and color variations of breastmilk.

5. Identify reasons for leakage of breastmilk, offering management recommendations.

6. Recognize the difference between two classifications of engorgement, offering recommendations for prevention and management.

7. Discuss possible causes of plugged ducts and provide recommendations for prevention and management.

8. Discuss possible causes of mastitis and provide recommendations for prevention and management.

9. Recognize signs and symptoms of an abscessed breast, offering recommendations for prevention and management.

10. Discuss the causes of a galactocele and management recommendations.

11. List signs of an overactive milk-ejection reflex and discuss management suggestions.

12. Discuss signs of an inhibited milk-ejection reflex, recognize possible causes, and offer management suggestions.

13. List factors contributing to an impaired milk supply and offer appropriate steps to assist the breastfeeding mother in increasing her milk supply.

OUTLINE

I. Candidiasis

    A. Causative factors

    B. Signs and symptoms
       1. The mother
       2. Spread among family members
       3. The infant

    C. Treatment

    D. Management suggestions

II. Herpes Simplex Virus

    A. Causative factors

    B. Management suggestions

III. Nipple Function Classification/Ungraspable Nipples

    A. Nipple differentiation
       1. The pinch test

    B. Treatment for dysfunction

    C. Management suggestions

IV. Nipple Discharges and/or Breastmilk Color Variations

    A. Causative factors and treatment
       1. Milky nipple discharge
       2. Bloody nipple discharge (sanguineous discharge)
       3. Multicolored, sticky nipple discharge
       4. Purulent nipple discharge
       5. Black-colored breastmilk
       6. Green- or pink-colored breastmilk

    B. Management suggestions

V. Leaking

    A. Causative factors and treatment

    B. Management suggestions

VI. Breast Engorgement

    A. Physiological engorgement

    B. Pathological engorgement

    C. Causative factors

    D. Treatment

    E. Management suggestions
       1. Ice flowers
       2. Cool cabbage-leaf compresses

VII. Plugged Ducts

    A. Signs and symptoms

    B. Causative factors

    C. Treatment

    D. Management suggestions

VIII. Mastitis

    A. Signs and symptoms

    B. Causative factors

    C. Treatment

    D. Management suggestions

IX. Abscessed Breast

    A. Signs and symptoms

    B. Causative factors

    C. Treatment

    D. Management suggestions

X. Galactocele

    A. Signs and symptoms

    B. Treatment

    C. Management suggestions

XI. Overactive Milk-Ejection Reflex

    A. Signs and symptoms

    B. Causative factors

    C. Treatment

    D. Management suggestions

XII. Impaired Milk-Ejection Reflex

    A. Signs and symptoms

    B. Causative factors

    C. Management suggestions

XIII. Inadequate Milk Supply

    A. Causative factors

    B. Management suggestions

PRE-TEST

For questions 1 to 9, choose the best answer.

1. Candidiasis
   A. can occur at any time during the breastfeeding relationship.
   B. occurs only in the newborn and early postpartum period.
   C. may appear only on the breastfeeding mother's nipples and the infant's oral cavity.
   D. Both A and C.

2. *Candida albicans*
   A. thrives on milk and warm, moist areas.
   B. is a common harmless organism that occurs normally in approximately one-half of the population.
   C. is another name for *Monilia albicans*.
   D. All of the above.

3. Predisposing factors for yeast infections include
   A. antibiotic therapy.
   B. oral contraceptive use.
   C. iron deficiency.
   D. All of the above.

4. A possible treatment for oral candidiasis found in infants is
   A. nystatin oral suspension.
   B. Monistat.
   C. Mycelex.
   D. Both A and C.

5. A mother with herpes simplex virus should be instructed to
   A. wean her infant immediately. Breastfeeding is contraindicated.
   B. wear gloves when breastfeeding her infant.
   C. interrupt breastfeeding from the affected breast until all lesions have healed and keep the breast pumped or expressed to maintain the milk supply.
   D. Both B and C.

6. Nipple discharges
   A. can be produced by endocrine processes or by local abnormalities.
   B. are all malignant.
   C. are all benign.
   D. Both A and B.

7. A spontaneous, sticky-type discharge that appears to be multicolored is
   A. caused by duct ectasia.
   B. comedomastitis.
   C. a breast abscess.
   D. Both A and B.

8. A bloody discharge during the lactation period may be due to
   A. trauma.
   B. carcinoma.
   C. vascular engorgement.
   D. All of the above.

9. Galactorrhea
    A. occurs bilaterally.
    B. is spontaneous milk discharge from multiple ducts in women of childbearing age.
    C. may be caused by an increased production of prolactin.
    D. Both B and C.
    E. All of the above.

For questions 10 to 15, choose the best answer from the following key:

    A. Physiological engorgement   **D. Mastitis**
    B. Pathological engorgement   **E. Abscessed breast**
    C. Plugged duct

10. May appear during the first week of the postpartum period. The mother may complain of warm, full, heavy breasts.

11. Mother may complain of a tender lump with possible redness in the area. She is afebrile.

12. Mother may complain of breast soreness and redness, flulike symptoms, and a temperature above 100.4°F.

13. May occur at any point during the breastfeeding relationship when the breasts are not emptied and milk accumulation in the breast is prolonged. The mother may complain of hot, swollen, red, and shiny breasts.

14. Mother complains of flulike symptoms, fever, and the infected site of the breast appears red, swollen, and is extremely tender to the touch.

15. A pus-filled area that does not respond to typical home treatment measures. Can form from an infection if treatment is delayed or inadequate.

For questions 16 to 20, choose the best answer from the following key:

    A. True   **B. False**

16. A galactocele is an enclosed sac containing substances ranging from milk to a thick, creamy, or oily substance. It is caused by an occlusion of a milk duct.

17. A mother who has an overactive milk-ejection reflex should limit nursings and pump the breasts prior to nursings.

18. A history of breast surgery or breast trauma may cause an impaired milk-ejection reflex.

19. A mother's milk supply may depend on the amount of infant demand and intake, or the frequency and duration of breastfeeding.

20. Breastfeeding is permitted with a breast abscess unless the abscess has ruptured into the ductile system.

Candidiasis

CAUSATIVE FACTORS

Candidiasis is an infection caused by a fungus of the genus *Candida*. An organism called *Candida albicans* is the most common etiologic agent, although involvement by other species is possible (Wei, 1988). *Candida albicans* thrives on milk and warm, moist areas, such as the breastfeeding infant's mouth, the breastfeeding mother's nipple area, lactiferous ducts, and a woman's vagina.

Candida albicans is a common, harmless organism that occurs normally in approximately one-half of the population; but under certain altered conditions, when usual defense mechanisms are disrupted, candida overgrowth on the skin and mucous membranes may cause an infection (De Coopman & Nehring, 1993; Johnston & Marcinak, 1990). Candida is an inhabitant of both normal and abnormal mucosal membranes like those lining the oral cavity and gastrointestinal tract.

Candida albicans—A small, oval, budding fungus that is the primary etiologic organism of candidiasis. Formerly referred to as *Monilia albicans*. It is a common and harmless organism found in mucous membranes, but under certain altered conditions may cause an infection.

Candidiasis—An infection of the skin or mucous membrane caused by a fungus of the genus *Candida (Monilia)*, especially *Candida albicans*.

Thrush—An infection of the mouth or throat caused by *Candida albicans* found especially in infants, young children, and immunocompromised individuals. It is characterized by the formation of white patches and ulcers, elevated temperature, and gastrointestinal inflammation.

Yeast—Any of several unicellular fungi of the genus *Saccharomyces* that reproduce by budding. They are capable of fermenting carbohydrates.

SIGNS AND SYMPTOMS

Candidiasis can occur at any time during the breastfeeding relationship. If the mother or infant is placed on antibiotic therapy during the breastfeeding period, candidiasis may develop because the antibiotics alter the normal flora (Amir, 1991). The nursing mother should be made aware of its signs and symptoms in order to initiate treatment as soon as possible if candidiasis does occur.

The Mother

Some or all of the following signs and symptoms occur in the breastfeeding mother who has candidiasis:

- Suddenly occurring, persistently painful nipples that do not respond to other treatment measures.

- Nipples that appear slightly pink to red in color, often accompanied by flaking, itching, or burning. Small white spots or small blisters may be seen on the nipples.
- Extremely painful nipples, and possibly areola, that often continues throughout a feeding and after a feeding session.
- Pains deep in the breasts that radiate up the breasts from the nipples during or between feedings, which may represent inflammation of the ducts with candidiasis (Amir, 1991).
- A vaginal, anal, or oral candida infection, angular cheilitis (inflammation of the lips at the corners), or paronychia (infection of marginal structures about the nail) (Amir, 1991).

Candidiasis can occur, and the infant be with or without obvious symptoms, while the mother is exhibiting typical signs and symptoms of the infection. A mother can be unaware of an occurring vaginal yeast infection because she may be asymptomatic, however (McCormack et al., 1985).

Predisposing factors for yeast infections include the following (Amir, 1991; De Coopman & Nehring, 1993; Hoover, 1992; Neville & Neifert, 1983; Wei, 1988):

- Diabetes mellitus
- Obesity
- Iron deficiency
- Steroidal drug use
- Oral contraceptive use
- Immunosuppressive drug use
- Diseases associated with immunological deficiency
- Antibiotic therapy
- Wearing tight jeans, pantyhose, a wet bathing suit, or wet nursing pads
- Diets high in artificial sweeteners, carbohydrates, or fermented food

Spread Among Family Members

Candida can be easily transferred between the mother and infant. The infant may acquire it during birth or it may even be transferred via the mother's hands or the infant's mouth (De Coopman & Nehring, 1993). The fungus may be transferred among family members if hygiene is poor. Older children may present with skin infections (Amir, 1991). If the mother has a candida infection, her sexual partner may present with a rash in the groin area (Amir, 1991).

The Infant

Candidiasis in the breastfed infant may appear on the perianal area or in the oral cavity and throat. Oral candidiasis may present in various clinical forms. Acute pseudomembranous candidiasis (thrush) is one of the common forms of oral candidiasis (Wei, 1988).

These are possible signs and symptoms occurring in the infant with candidiasis:

- A diaper rash that appears as fiery red sores or sore-looking pustules appearing on the infant's perianal area.

- Oral candidiasis may occur on any mucosal surface—the tongue, gums, cheeks, palate, throat, and floor of the mouth. It appears as a white, creamy, soft plaque, resembling milk curds, that cannot be easily washed off. If this pseudomembrane surface is removed, it leaves an erythematous surface (Wei, 1988).
- The infant may begin refusing the breast or appear fussy and reluctant to breastfeed due to soreness of the mouth (Hoover, 1992).

TREATMENT

If candidiasis is suspected, the client should be referred to a physician or a public health nurse practitioner for diagnosis and simultaneous treatment of both her infant and herself. It is extremely important that both mother and infant (and any other affected family members) be treated, or they will continue to reinfect each other. Encourage the mother to continue the medications until the entire course is completed because candidiasis may reappear if treatment is stopped prematurely.

Candidiasis can invade the ductal system of the breast and should be suspected when the lactating mother complains of burning or stinging pains radiating up the breast. If candidiasis of the duct system is confirmed, treatment with a systemic antifungal agent may also be needed (Lawrence, 1989). Once treatment has begun, relief may be noticed within approximately 24 hours to 5 days. Sometimes symptoms may worsen before they begin to improve.

A common treatment is the use of antifungal medications like nystatin (Mycostatin) suspension for the infant's oral cavity and nystatin ointment, clotrimazole (Gyne-Lotrimin, Mycelex), and miconizole (Monistat) for the mother's nipples and areolas. Gentian violet is an alternative treatment sometimes used in place of these; it works adequately; however, there are potential risk factors associated with its use. A possible problem with gentian violet use is blistering of the infant's oral cavity. This could occur with overusing the gentian violet or from not diluting it sufficiently during preparation (Utter, 1992). Mycolog is a medication that is sometimes prescribed for treatment of the infant's perianal area. If the infection has progressed to a more moderate stage, a systemic antifungal medication like fluconazole (Diflucan) or ketoconazole (Nizoral) may be indicated. Once the diagnosis of candidiasis has been confirmed, the mother should take precautions to help prevent the spread of infection and to prevent the infection from reoccurring.

MANAGEMENT SUGGESTIONS FOR THE MOTHER AND INFANT WITH CANDIDIASIS

Instruct the mother to do the following if candida infection is present:

1. Continue breastfeeding. Weaning should not be indicated. In the cases of severe nipple pain, the mother may desire to hand-express her breast for a brief period before putting the infant back to the breast.
2. Wash hands frequently, using good handwashing techniques. Cleanliness may help prevent recurrence.

3. The mother should contact her physician or public health nurse practitioner for diagnosis and treatment.

4. The breastfeeding mother and infant must be treated simultaneously with an antifungal medication.

5. If the infection recurs after treatment, all family members may need to be treated. Older children may present with skin infections/rashes. The mother's sexual partner may also be infected, which may be the cause of the reinfection. The sexual partner may present with a groin rash (Amir, 1991).

6. The mother, infant, and other infected family members must complete the full course of medication to prevent recurrence.

7. If oral suspension of nystatin is prescribed, the mother should be instructed on proper application. The medication should be kept in contact with the oral mucosa for several minutes before being swallowed. In infants, application can be with a swab. Medication should not be squeezed or dropped into the infant's mouth because that may induce the infant to swallow it prematurely.

8. The breastfeeding mother should be treated with an antifungal intravaginal preparation if she has a vaginal yeast infection.

9. If the infant uses rubber teats, pacifiers/dummies, or teething toys, they should be boiled daily, then discarded at the end of one week's time and new ones used.

10. Other toys that the infant puts in his mouth should be cleaned frequently with hot, soapy water to help prevent reinfection and spread to other children.

11. The mother's nipple area should be kept as dry as possible. Nursing pads should be changed at each feeding, at a minimum. The mother should not express breastmilk onto the nipples after breastfeeding because the fungi ferment carbohydrates. Instead, after feedings, the nipple, areola, and infant's mouth should be rinsed with water to remove any residual milk.

12. If the mother is using a breast pump, encourage proper cleaning of all pump parts (per pump instructions), including daily boiling of the parts coming into contact with breastmilk. The parts should be washed with hot, soapy water and boiled for 20 minutes once a day until the infection is no longer evident.

13. The mother should wash her bras and panties and the infant's cloth diapers (if used) daily in hot water until treatment has been completed (Hoover, 1992). The mother should wear 100% cotton underpants and bras and use 100% cotton diapers on the infant. Disposable diaper use is not recommended if the infant's perianal area is infected with candida.

Herpes Simplex Virus

CAUSATIVE FACTORS

Herpes simplex virus (HSV) infection during the neonatal period is severe. Contamination of the neonate may occur during vaginal births when the mothers are infected and have active genital herpes lesions. Breastfeeding is not contraindicated for the mother with genital herpes, with careful hygienic handling of the infant to prevent the cross-spread (World Health Organization, 1990).

If transmission of HSV occurs during the breastfeeding period, it is most likely through direct contact with a lesion on the breast (Riordan & Auerbach, 1993). While HSV can be cultured from breastmilk, spreading this way is a rare occurrence. According to a 1979 published report, HSV/Type I may have possibly been acquired by an infant via breastmilk during the postpartum period. Careful examination revealed that the only possible source of the virus was the mother's breastmilk (Dunkle, Schmidt, & O'Conner, 1979).

Little information on HSV and breastfeeding is available; but because the population of breastfeeding women is increasing, as well as the known cases of HSV, health-care professionals must become aware of the implications of HSV for the breastfeeding duo. The majority of HSV cases are HSV I, fever blisters or cold sores, or HSV II, genital herpes (AAP & ACOG, 1992). Breastfeeding is allowed when the mother has no vesicular herpetic lesions on the breast area and all active cutaneous lesions are covered (AAP & ACOG, 1992).

The American Academy of Pediatrics (AAP) Committee on the Fetus and Newborn and the Committee on Infectious Disease presented recommendations in 1980 regarding HSV. They recommend that, with extreme care paid to good hygiene, the mother and infant not be separated when the mother has an outbreak of genital lesions. If the lactating mother has a lesion on the breast, breastfeeding is contraindicated and should not resume until the lesion has healed and been cultured negative (Neville & Neifert, 1983). All lesions that are present should be covered sufficiently to prevent cross-contamination. Breastfeeding from the unaffected breast may continue with extreme emphasis placed on good hygiene routines. Good handwashing techniques, clean covering, and restricted fondling and kissing of the infant during a period of outbreak should be encouraged until lesions are healed (Lawrence, 1989; World Health Organization, 1990).

It is extremely important that the breastfeeding mother with an HSV lesion on her breast be instructed on maintaining her milk supply in the affected breast. She should express milk during this period of healing. If the mother's breast pump or hand come into contact with a lesion while expressing, the milk should be discarded and not given to the infant, because it is possible that it is contaminated with the virus. The mother should immediately wash her hands and sterilize the pump parts.

Herpes simplex virus during the newborn period has been shown to be severely harmful, and even fatal, for infected infants. Pregnant or lactating women should consult their physician for diagnosis and advise if HSV infection is suspected. After obtaining a culture from the lesion, confirmed diagnosis can usually be made within a very few days (Lawrence, 1989). Acyclovir is used to treat HSV infection, although use is usually limited during pregnancy (AAP & ACOG, 1992) to the presence of life-threatening HSV infection (encephalitis, pneumonitis, hepatitis). Acyclovir therapy in neonatal units is common. Breastmilk levels have been reported to produce no overt side effects in infants and the AAP considers acyclovir compatible with breastfeeding (American Academy of Pediatrics, 1994; Meyer et al., 1988; Taddio, Klein, & Koren, 1994).

MANAGEMENT SUGGESTIONS FOR THE LACTATING MOTHER WITH HSV LESION ON BREAST

Instruct the mother to do the following if an outbreak of HSV lesions occurs:

1. Contact a physician for diagnosis and treatment if HSV is suspected.

2. If HSV lesions are on the nipple or areola of the breast, advise against breastfeeding on the affected breast until lesions are healed. Breastfeeding may continue on the unaffected breast. If the mother has oral HSV lesions, she should avoid kissing the infant until lesions are crusted and dried. If the mother has genital HSV lesions, she may breastfeed provided she uses a clean barrier to prevent infant contact with lesions or any infectious materials, such as her underclothes and lochia-soiled materials.

3. If breastfeeding is interrupted for a period while lesions are healing, instruct the mother on expression of breastmilk. If waiting for a confirmation of HSV diagnosis, instruct the mother to express and discard the breastmilk from the affected side or sides. If a breast pump is used on a breast with a lesion, it should not also be used on the unaffected breast.

4. Whenever HSV lesions are present, instruct on clean covering of the area, good handwashing techniques, meticulous hygiene measures, and careful handling of the infant until lesions are healed, to help prevent cross-contamination. There is no indication for the breastfeeding mother to wear gloves while breastfeeding her infant.

5. If any member of the family has an outbreak of HSV, the person should avoid close contact with the infant and use good hygiene measures.

6. The breastfeeding mother's sexual partner should not kiss her breasts during a HSV outbreak (Mohrbacher & Stock, 1991).

Nipple Function Classification/Ungraspable Nipples

NIPPLE DIFFERENTIATION

During the prenatal period, breast examination should be performed, including careful inspection of the nipple area. Just as variation occurs in breast size, shape, and symmetry among women, so do types of nipples.

The Pinch Test

The pinch test is a brief test that checks the nipple's ability to protract. The areola is grasped, beyond the base of the nipple, between the thumb and forefinger. It is then compressed, or pinched, together and quickly released. Observation should be based on the reaction of the stimulated nipple (see Figure 2C–1):

    A. Protracting normal nipple
    B. Moderate-to-severe retraction
    C. Inverted-appearing nipple when compressed using pinch test will either invert farther inward or protract forward (upper right)
    D. True inversion; nipple inverts further (lower right).

Figure 2C–1

Nipple classification.

Source: Diane Davis, artist. Reprinted with permission. Concept from Riordan, J, Auerbach, KG (1993). *Breastfeeding and Human Lactation.* Boston: Jones and Bartlett.

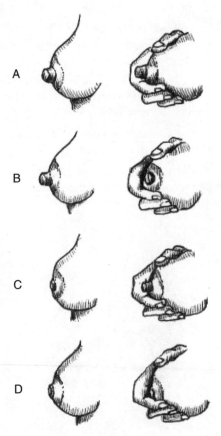

According to Riordan and Auerbach (1993), the following are classifications of nipple function:

Complete—The nipple does not respond to manual pressure because adhesions bind the nipple inward; very rarely there is congenital absence of the nipple.

Inversion—On visual inspection, all or part of the nipple is drawn inward within the folds of the areola.

Minimal—An infant with a strong suck exerts sufficient pressure to pull the nipple forward. A weak or premature infant may have difficulties at first.

Moderate to Severe—Retracts to a level even with or behind the surrounding areola. Intervention is helpful to stretch the nipple outward and improve protractability.

Protraction—Nipple moves forward; considered a normal functional response. No special interventions are needed.

Retraction—Instead of protracting, the nipple moves inward.

Simple—The nipple moves outward to protraction with manual pressure or when cold (pseudoinversion).

TREATMENT FOR DYSFUNCTION

Dysfunction of the nipple can occur bilaterally or unilaterally. If dysfunction is unilateral, the mother may note a definite preference for one breast over the other. The infant can adapt to the type of nipple given, but may require extra assistance and patience if the mother's nipple is flat, dimpled, or inverted. The newborn infant must be able to draw the mother's nipple into his or her mouth for sucking. Some infants may consistently refuse to breastfeed on the dysfunctional nipple, and the mother may decide to continue breastfeeding on one side only. This is acceptable, but stress frequent breastfeeding in order to provide an adequate milk supply for the infant. Other mothers object to the disparity in the size of the breasts that develops when only one breast is used and prefer to pump the other breast, storing the milk for future outings.

Treatment of flat and inverted nipples should begin prenatally to help prevent a frustrated infant and mother when the breastfeeding relationship begins. As soon as the nipples have been inspected and a dysfunctional nipple noted, client education should begin and plans for nipple treatment discussed. Breast shells, also referred to as milk cups, are a treatment option that should be considered. Breast shells are plastic, vented domes that are worn in the bra cups. They have two different types of backs that fit on the domes. One type aids in the healing of sore nipples; the other is a ring that assists in pulling the nipple outward by providing a constant, gentle pressure around the nipple area. The breast shells can be worn during the last trimester of pregnancy or between feedings during the postpartum period.

During the prenatal period, rough nipple manipulation is not recommended because it can be dangerous and is very rarely successful. Uterine contractions

(Elliot & Flaherty, 1983) and damage to the Montgomery's tubercles could occur. Nipple rolling during the postpartum period may be extremely helpful. Nipple rolling prior to a feeding may help the nipple to protract and assist the infant to latch easier. Also, using a pump to pull out the nipple before feedings may protract the nipple.

In the postpartum period, some have found Hoffman's exercises helpful (see Figure 2C–2). Hoffman's exercises were developed for separating adhesions at the nipple's base that may be causing the nipple to invert. It involves placing the thumbs or forefingers of each hand on opposite sides of the nipple's base and stretching outward from the nipple. The fingers should be rotated to different positions, and the exercise repeated. Some lactation consultants no longer recommend using Hoffman's exercises and breast shells based on the results of one study where no benefit was shown (Alexander et al., 1993).

In an article published in the *Journal of Human Lactation*, a homemade device (see Figure 2C–3) for drawing out inverted nipples using a syringe was described (Kesaree, 1993, p. 28):

1. Remove the plunger and cut off the nozzle-end of a disposable 10 ml syringe barrel.
2. Reinsert the syringe plunger into the barrel from the cut end, so it is away from the mother's nipple.
3. Apply the syringe device to the nipple and pull gently on the plunger to create suction. The nipple will evert into the syringe.

A new product by Maternal Concepts—the Evert-It™—has recently been marketed to use in cases of nipple retraction or inversion. There are no reports of clinical trials to determine its effectiveness.

Figure 2C–2

Hoffman's exercises.
Source: Diane Davis, artist.
Reprinted with permission.

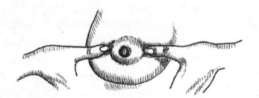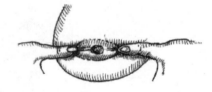

Figure 2C–3

Device made from syringe for drawing out inverted nipples.

Source: Kesaree, N, et al. (1993). Treatment of inverted nipples using a disposable syringe. *J Hum Lact*, 9:28. Reprinted with permission of Human Sciences Press.

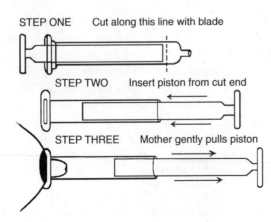

STEP ONE   Cut along this line with blade

STEP TWO   Insert piston from cut end

STEP THREE   Mother gently pulls piston

Only as a last resort should a nipple shield made of a thin silicone material be used. Instructions must be given to the mother on proper use. After the mother experiences a milk-ejection reflex, the nipple shield should be removed from the breast, and the infant latched directly onto the breast. Often, first attempts to remove the nipple shield are not successful, and the nipple shield must be used for a period of time before the infant is able to latch on without it. During this time, the counselor must provide follow-up to weigh the infant and determine the adequacy of the feeds with the nipple shield. All the hazards of nipple-shield use should be discussed with the mother prior to use, with the mother verbalizing her understanding. Use of the nipple shield and the reason for use should be well documented in notes (Minchin, 1989).

MANAGEMENT SUGGESTIONS FOR THE MOTHER WITH UNGRASPABLE NIPPLES

Instruct the mother with ungraspable nipples to do the following:

1. Inspect the breasts, paying close attention to the nipples, during the prenatal period. Observe the reaction of the stimulated nipple after performing the pinch test (see Figure 2C–4).
2. If a dysfunctional nipple is noted, discuss treatment options (breast shells, Hoffman's exercises, devices to evert the nipple, nipple shields for feeding).
3. Provide specifics on the treatment devices—breast shells, disposable syringe (or Materna Evert-It), and nipple shields (from Garrett & Ashworth, 1996).

Pinch Test

- Wash hands.
- With forefinger and thumb just beyond the nipple base, compress or squeeze the areola one time.
- Observe nipple reaction to pinch test.

Figure 2C–4

The pinch test.

Source: Spangler, A (1995). *Breastfeeding: A Parent's Guide*, p. 26. Reprinted with permission of author and Childbirth Graphics.

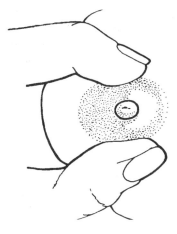

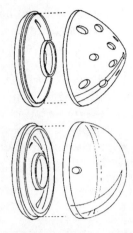

Figure 2C–5
Breast shells used for the treatment of flat or inverted nipples.
Source: Diane Davis, artist.

Breast Shells

- Gradually increase the time that breast shells are worn.
- Choose the bra size that will accommodate using a breast shell without making the bra too tight, in order to prevent possible problems with plugged ducts.
- Choose breast shells that have well-vented domes. Avoid shells that have only one or very few holes—they tend to seal in moisture, which could lead to tender nipples or an infection (see Figure 2C–5).
- Do not wear breast shells excessively or while sleeping—they can cause problems with mastitis and plugged ducts. If redness or swelling of the breast is noted, discontinue using the breast shells. After several days, the mother may consider wearing them again occasionally and for shorter periods of time.
- Breastmilk that has collected in the breast shells should be discarded and not saved for baby; it may be harboring bacteria.
- Sterilize the breast shells on a weekly basis; wash them with hot, soapy water daily. If the mother has been diagnosed with a candida infection on the nipple or areola area, suggest daily sterilizing.

Hoffman's Exercises

- Place thumbs or forefingers opposite each other on either side of the nipple.
- Gently draw thumbs or forefingers away from the nipple.
- Repeat with fingers above and below the nipple.
- Do numerous times each day.

Disposable Syringe or Materna Evert-It

- Use on each breast prior to feeding.
- Rinse with hot water after each feeding and clean with hot, soapy water daily.
- Discontinue use if damage to the nipple occurs.

Nipple Shields

- Choose one made of thin silicone material that will accommodate the mother's nipple and areolar tissue and the infant's mouth (see example in Figure 2C–6).
- Use expressed breastmilk to wet the nipple and areola.
- Invert the brim of the shield as if you are going to turn it inside out.
- When the diameter of the inside of the shield brim matches the diameter of the nipple, place the inside of the crown over the nipple.
- Then smooth the brim of the shield over the areola and hold it in place.
- The edge of the crown will press into the areola; so hold the brim against the areola, and tease the crown out from the breast. Suction will then pull the nipple forward into the shield.
- The shield may then be taped securely in place, if desired.
- Shape the breast, and apply slight pressure on the top of the shield's brim during latch-on.

Figure 2C–6

One type of nipple shield.

Source: Product of Medela, Inc. (McHenry, IL). Reprinted with permission.

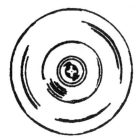
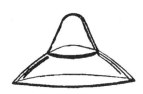

- Use at the beginning of the feeding for 1 to 2 minutes, or until the nipple has everted and the first milk-ejection reflex has occurred.
- Break the suction of the infant, and remove the infant from the breast.
- Remove the nipple shield, and re-attach the infant to the breast.

Nipple Discharges and/or Breastmilk Color Variations

CAUSATIVE FACTORS AND TREATMENT

Pathologic breast secretions can be produced by endocrine processes or possibly by local abnormalities (Tabar et al., 1974). The majority of nipple discharges are caused by benign lesions in the lactating mother's breast; however, all discharges deserve careful observation because of the possibility of a malignancy. Physician referral is indicated to determine the cause of nipple discharge (Lawrence, 1989).

Cases have been reported of infants abruptly refusing to feed on a breast, rejecting the milk, and subsequently a malignant mass being discovered in the breast (Goldsmith, 1974). Factors making the breastmilk from a breast containing a carcinoma undesirable to the infant have not been determined. If a breastfeeding mother discovers a mass in the breast and at the same time the infant is presenting a milk-rejection sign, physician referral is indicated (Goldsmith, 1974).

Milky Nipple Discharge

The woman who complains of continued bilateral lactation that appears as a milky discharge after she has quit breastfeeding for more than three months is often diagnosed with galactorrhea. Galactorrhea is a bilaterally occurring, spontaneous milk discharge from multiple ducts in women of childbearing age. Galactorrhea may be caused by an increased production of prolactin (hyperprolactinemia), direct action of the pituitary gland, or inadequate hypothalamic inhibition of the pituitary gland (Leis, 1988). Other possible causes include Chiari–Frommel syndrome; Forbes–Albright syndrome; Ahumada–Del Castilla syndrome; pituitary adenomas; hypothyroidism; thyrotoxicosis; and patients taking medications like phenothiazines, tricyclic antidepressants, rauwolfia alkaloids, methyldopa, and oral contraceptives (Leis, 1988). Physician referral is indicated for a specific diagnosis.

Bloody Nipple Discharge (Sanguineous Discharge)

Most bleeding from the nipple is benign. O'Callaghan (1981) reported on cases of red–brown or rusty-colored milk discharge appearing in 32 women. Appearing as early as the second trimester of pregnancy, it was associated with antenatal breast expression in more than one-half of the women.

A bloody discharge during the lactation period may be caused by trauma to the breast area or possibly from vascular engorgement. In the absence of nipple trauma, papillomas or fibrocystic disease have also been known to also cause a bloody-type discharge from the lactating breast (Lawrence, 1989). In most cases, the bleeding stops on its own without treatment; however, if it recurs or persists, physician referral is indicated (Riordan & Auerbach, 1993). Bloody discharge from the nipple can indicate carcinoma; so it is important that the client see a physician to determine the cause (Lawrence, 1989; Tabar, Marton, & Kadas, 1974).

Multicolored, Sticky Nipple Discharge

A complaint of a spontaneous, sticky-type discharge that appears to be multicolored is most often caused by duct ectasia (dilatation of the ducts), also called comedomastitis. The discharge is commonly greenish, but may also appear yellow, white, gray, and brown (Leis, 1988). A mother with duct ectasia may also complain of an itching, burning pain and swelling of the nipple and areola area of the breast. A progression of the disease may produce a mass (Leis, 1988; Lawrence, 1989). If a mass develops or discharge becomes bloody, surgical excision of the mass may be indicated (Leis, 1988). Physician referral is indicated for a specific diagnosis.

Purulent Nipple Discharge

A unilateral, spontaneous, purulent discharge can be caused by an infection, predominantly a staphylococcal infection. Symptoms include nipple or breast tenderness and inflammation or possibly the formation of an abscess. This type of discharge may be seen in patients presenting with puerperal mastitis, chronic lactation mastitis, or an abscess (Leis, 1988). Purulent discharge from the nipple should be treated with an antibiotic. Physician referral is indicated for a specific diagnosis.

Black-Colored Breastmilk

A semisynthetic derivative of tetracycline, minocycline hydrochloride (Minocin), has been found in the breastmilk of women taking this drug and has been associated with black milk. Basler and Lynch (1985) report a case of a woman taking minocycline hydrochloride for the treatment of severe acne for four years presenting with black milk during galactorrhea. Physician referral is indicated for a specific diagnosis.

Green- or Pink-Colored Breastmilk

Foods containing red and yellow dyes, such as some orange sodas, have been linked to reports of pink- or orange-colored breast milk. Several cases of green-colored breastmilk have been shown to be the result of the ingestion of natural vitamins from health-food sources, sports drinks, or products derived from seaweed (Lawrence, 1989). Physician referral is indicated for a specific diagnosis.

MANAGEMENT SUGGESTIONS FOR THE MOTHER WITH NIPPLE DISCHARGE OR COLORED BREASTMILK

Follow these guidelines when counseling the mother experiencing nipple discharge or a variation in breastmilk color:

1. Physician referral is indicated if there is any abnormality.
2. Strongly encourage self-examination of the breasts. The optimal time for examining the lactating breast is following a breastfeeding session, when the breasts are least full, and at the end of the menstrual cycle. Changes in

the breast are more easily recognized by the women who perform breast self-exams on a regular basis. While it is rare, breast cancer in pregnant and lactating women does occur. It is estimated that 1–2% of all breast cancers occur among pregnant and lactating women (Schwartz, 1982).

3. Purulent discharge from the nipple should be treated with an antibiotic.

Leaking

CAUSATIVE FACTORS AND TREATMENT

Many lactating women leak breastmilk, and this is considered part of the normal breastfeeding process. Leaking most often occurs during the early weeks of the breastfeeding relationship, when the breasts are full, or in association with the milk-ejection reflex, such as leaking from the opposite breast during a breastfeeding session, when hearing a crying infant, or during sexual arousal.

If leaking occurs during an inconvenient time for the mother, exerting gentle pressure on the nipple toward the chest wall can help stop it. The mother can do this discreetly by folding her arms across her chest, as in a relaxed position, or applying pressure with a finger to the nipple. If the mother tends to leak during sexual arousal, suggest she nurse beforehand to empty the breasts. This may not actually stop leaking from occurring, but may decrease the amount. A new product, *blis* (Breast Leakage Inhibitor System), from Prolac, Inc. (Skaneateles, NY), provides gentle pressure to the nipple to minimize leaking. The safety and effectiveness of this product have not been published.

Extreme, inappropriate, or continued leaking is symptomatic of galactorrhea. Galactorrhea is milk secretion that continues for longer than 3 to 6 months after weaning or a nonphysiological milk secretion that occurs independent of lactation (Vorherr, Vorherr, McConnell, et al., 1974). Drugs that interfere with dopamine release may contribute to excessive milk secretion because dopamine inhibits prolactin. Use of intrauterine devices containing copper have also been reported as possible causes of abnormal milk secretion (Horn & Scott, 1969).

Possible pathological causes of galactorrhea during the lactation process include pituitary adenomas, Chiari–Frommel syndrome, Forbes–Albright syndrome, Ahumada–Del Castilla syndrome (Leis, 1988), hypothyroidism (Vorherr, 1974), and thyrotoxicosis (Lawrence, 1989). Medications like phenothiazines, tricyclic antidepressants, rauwolfia alkaloids, methyldopa, and oral contraceptives have been reported to cause galactorrhea (Leis, 1988). Any female presenting with persistent and extreme secretion of milk should seek medical attention.

MANAGEMENT SUGGESTIONS FOR THE MOTHER WHO IS LEAKING

Guidelines for assisting the mother who has problems with leaking include:

1. Offer understanding and encouragement to the mother who is experiencing leaking.
2. Instruct her on ways to stop or minimize the leaking if it occurs during an inappropriate time, such as applying firm, yet gentle pressure to the breast/nipple area in the direction of the chest wall.
3. Instruct on nipple care and changing bra pads when they are damp.

4. Offer suggestions on clothing that may not show obvious signs of leaking. Suggest wearing light-colored clothing rather than dark when possible, and encourage clothing with patterns/prints. Suggest that the working mother take a jacket or extra blouse to work.

5. Suggest breastfeeding prior to sexual activity.

6. Find out if the woman is taking any medication that may possibly be contributing to excessive milk production.

7. Encourage any female presenting with galactorrhea to seek medical attention—it may be symptomatic of a more serious problem.

8. Tell her about the *blis* product.

Breast Engorgement

Whether engorgement is or is not a normal part of lactogenesis is the subject of much debate and confusion. To assist in understanding this phenomenon, engorgement can be classified in two ways: physiological engorgement and pathological engorgement (Shrago, 1991).

PHYSIOLOGICAL ENGORGEMENT

Physiological engorgement appears during the first week of the postpartum period as lactogenesis occurs. The mother may complain of warm, full, heavy breasts. Congestion and edema of breast tissues as blood and other fluids accumulate, incorporated with the increased milk volume in the alveoli, lactiferous ducts, and lactiferous sinuses, are characteristic of physiological engorgement as lactation begins. Due to the firmness caused by engorgement of the breast and areola tissue, the infant may present with an improper latch-on, which leads to sore nipples and inadequate emptying of the lactiferous sinuses, which may in turn lead to more severe problems like pathological engorgement and a frustrated, unsatisfied infant (Shrago, 1991).

PATHOLOGICAL ENGORGEMENT

Pathological engorgement can occur at any point during the breastfeeding relationship when the breasts are not emptied and milk accumulation in the breast is prolonged (Shrago, 1991). The mother may complain that her breasts are hot, swollen, hard, and possibly red and shiny. She may have an elevated temperature. Unrelieved engorgement can eventually cause decreased milk supply due to milk stasis of the lactiferous ducts, which causes the secretory cells of the alveoli to flatten and discontinue milk production. Frequent emptying of the breasts beginning in the early postpartum period and continuing throughout the breastfeeding relationship, combined with proper infant positioning and latch-on, is significant in reducing the occurrence of pathological engorgement. Prevention is the best cure.

CAUSATIVE FACTORS

The possible causes of engorgement, according to Moon and Humenick (1989) and Lauwers and Woessner (1990), follow:

- Missed breastfeedings
- Delayed breastfeedings
- Infrequent breastfeedings
- Restricted or shortened breastfeedings
- Breast not emptied at breastfeedings
- Complementary feeds used

- Supplementary feeds used
- Inadequate milk-ejection reflex
- Baby is sleepy or unenthusiastic about nursing

TREATMENT

With aggressive treatment measures, engorgement may be relieved within a 24-hour time frame. Comfort measures for engorgement are frequent emptying of the breasts through unlimited access by the infant, every 1 to 2 hours. Do not limit the amount of time the infant spends at the breast; encourage at least 15- to 20-minute sessions.

Measures that enhance the milk-ejection reflex may prove helpful in assisting with the milk flow in engorgement. Applying warm, moist heat to the breasts or taking a warm shower prior to breastfeeding may prove helpful for the early stages of physiologic engorgement but are not recommended for pathological engorgement. Encourage massaging the breasts prior to and during a breastfeeding session if the mother can tolerate it. Types of breast massage include fingertip massage, diamond–hand position massage, parallel hand massage, and the Japanese method of breast massage. Brief manual expression of milk prior to nursing softens the areola and makes an adequate latch-on easier to achieve. Massage and hand expression are covered in more detail in Chapter 3 in this module.

After a breastfeeding session, the mother should express milk to further empty the breasts; expression helps to correct the stasis of milk and provides maternal comfort. Applying ice to the breasts after a nursing session may help relieve swelling and provide comfort. Ice should always be used if the flow of milk is impeded by swollen breasts. Using heat in these situations only aggravates the problem. Some women complain that the weight of the ice cubes is uncomfortable. Submersing the breasts in a basin of ice water or using crushed ice (a bag of frozen peas also works) may prove a comforting alternative.

MANAGEMENT SUGGESTIONS FOR ENGORGEMENT

Follow these guidelines to assist the mother with discomfort from engorgement:

1. Frequent, on-demand breastfeeding, every one to two hours around the clock. Allow the infant unlimited time at the breast. Frequent nursings help prevent milk stasis.

2. Prior to breastfeeding, apply warm, moist compresses to the breasts, soak the breasts in warm water, or shower for approximately 10 to 15 minutes. This may facilitate the milk-ejection reflex. This suggestion is advised only for the early stages of physiological engorgement.

3. Gentle, manual expression can soften the areola of the breast for appropriate infant attachment.

4. Electric-piston breast pumps on a low setting may be used, if necessary, to soften the engorged areola so the infant can latch on to the breast appropriately. Using a breast pump to try to alleviate the engorgement pro-

duces little breastmilk and could possibly cause trauma to a breast that is excessively vascular (Lawrence, 1989).

5. Gently massage the breasts before and during a nursing session if the mother can tolerate it.

6. Have the breastfeeding mother vary the nursing positions used to help promote drainage of lactiferous sinuses and lactiferous ducts.

7. Apply ice to the breasts following a nursing session for approximately 20 minutes. In cases of extreme engorgement, apply the clean, inner leaves of a cabbage as a compress; the leaves should be changed upon wilting or after two hours. Evaluate the breasts for reduced swelling and enhanced milk flow with each change of cabbage leaves until desired results are obtained (Rosier, 1988).

8. Encourage wearing a well-fitted bra for support and avoiding underwire styles.

9. Advise the breastfeeding mother to call with symptoms of a temperature greater than 100.6°F, or localized pain, chills, body aches, or other flulike symptoms. Breastfeeding is not contraindicated if the breastfeeding mother has an elevated temperature.

Ice Flowers

Marmet and Shell (1981) have successfully used "ice flowers" to treat engorgement. Ice flowers can be made by placing crushed ice in three small plastic sandwich bags and sealing each one. Each plastic bag should be double-bagged by placing it inside another plastic bag. Again, seal each one individually. Each bag of ice is considered a "petal." Tie the three petals together. Place a towel on the breasts and apply the ice flower, with each petal covering a different area of the breast. Never place the ice flower directly on the breast.

Cool Cabbage-Leaf Compresses

Another remedy for pathological engorgement is the application of cabbage-leaf compresses to the breasts. This method is an ancient remedy attributed to Chinese or continental European settlers in Australia's early history. Case studies using this technique successfully have been reported (Rosier, 1988). In a randomized, controlled study of 120 women, 60 women were advised to give standard care for engorgement: heat, massage, and breastmilk expression. The other 60 were advised to apply cold cabbage leaves to their breasts. Although the researchers were not able to confirm a direct effect of cabbage leaves on breast engorgement, no harmful effects were found. The researchers did find that when breastfeeding rates at six-weeks postpartum were compared, 76% of the experimental group continued to breastfeed exclusively while only 58% in the standard care group did. Also, fewer in the experimental group discontinued breastfeeding before eight days (Nikoden et al., 1993).

For severe cases of engorgement, clean, inner cabbage leaves can be substituted for ice at the completion of a breastfeeding or pumping session. Change the leaves after two hours or upon wilting. Extreme caution should be used when recommending the use of cabbage compresses because extended use has been shown to suppress lactation. Make clients considering this technique aware of the foulsmelling odor of the wilted leaves. Avoid this technique if the patient has ever shown any type of sensitivity to cabbage.

Plugged Ducts

SIGNS AND SYMPTOMS

Plugged ducts are also referred to as blocked ducts, caked breasts, or the clogging of milk. If the breastfeeding mother complains of a tender or sore lump, with possible redness in the area of the breast that often follows the direction of a duct, and is afebrile, suspect a plugged duct.

CAUSATIVE FACTORS

Causes of plugged ducts include stress, poor nutrition, inadequate emptying of the breasts, missed feedings, or areas of pressure exerted on the breast by external sources (such as wearing a bra that is too tight or with underwire support, always sleeping in one position) (Maher, 1988). White granules believed to be casein micelles and hydroxyapatite form particulate lumps in the breastmilk of some women and may be responsible for obstructing milk ducts (Australian Lactation Consultant Association, 1992). Strings of fatty-looking material have been described by mothers (Minchin, 1985) and may be caused by inspissated milk.

TREATMENT

A blister at the end of the duct on the nipple often accompanies a plugged duct. Sometimes the blister can be drained, but most often (until the duct is cleared) it refills with milk. Occasionally, a sterile-needle aspiration is necessary to draw out the coagulated milk. [Note that in some cases the blister is not associated with a plugged duct but with sore nipples. It signals the maturation of basal cells as epithelial cells migrate across the surface of a skin fissure and healing occurs. These blisters should not be aspirated.]

The breastfeeding mother should be encouraged to begin efforts to remove the plug as soon as symptoms are noted in order to prevent further complications. If the suspected plug does not respond to treatment measures, contact a physician for further diagnosis and treatment.

MANAGEMENT SUGGESTIONS FOR PLUGGED DUCTS

Instruct the mother with plugged ducts to do the following:

1. Continue frequent breastfeeding sessions—at least every two to three hours. Infrequent breastfeeding can cause increased discomfort and possibly lead to a breast abscess.

2. Applying moist, warm heat to the affected area combined with gentle massage just above the affected area, moving downward toward the nipple area, promotes milk flow and circulation. Gentle massage during a warm shower and leaning over a basin of warm water are also effective.

3. Nurse from the breast with the suspected plug first. If the breast is too tender and the mother is experiencing extreme discomfort, she may try initiating nursing on the unaffected breast first to allow the milk-ejection reflex to occur on the affected breast without the pressure of the infant's sucking.

4. Nurse with the infant's nose pointing towards the suspected plug at the beginning of the feeding, changing positions when appropriate to ensure emptying of all breast areas.

5. During nursing sessions, continue to use moist, warm compresses and massage to the affected area to promote the release of the plug. Warmth promotes vasodilation, an increase in circulation, and an increase in lymph flow.

6. Apply ice to the breasts between breastfeeding sessions to help reduce inflammation.

7. Encourage maternal rest.

8. Look for the possible etiology, and offer suggestions to help prevent recurrence.

9. If the suspected plugged duct does not respond to treatment measures, contact a physician for further diagnosis and treatment.

Mastitis

SIGNS AND SYMPTOMS

If the breastfeeding mother complains of flulike symptoms, including a temperature greater than 38.4°C or 101°F and feeling fatigued, mastitis should be suspected. The area of the breast that is infected may appear red, tender, and hot to the touch.

CAUSATIVE FACTORS

Mastitis is classified as noninfective and infective. Noninfective mastitis is an infection of the breast tissue that is often caused by pressure internally or externally, which causes stasis of milk, preventing the proper drainage of milk. Other nonpathogenic causes of mastitis have been hypothesized, including fatigue, stress, untreated engorgement or plugged duct, breast trauma, milk stasis, malnutrition, breast constriction (i.e., tight clothing or bras), and vigorous upper arm exercise (Dilts, 1985; Riordan & Nichols, 1990).

Infective mastitis may be preceded by nipple breakdown, which allows a pathogen to enter the body. The usual site of entry of infectious pathogens is through the lactiferous sinuses, through fissures in the nipple to the periductal lymphatics, or possibly through hematogenous spread (Lawrence, 1994; Niebyl, 1978). Staphylococcus aureus is the most common infecting organism in mastitis. Escherichia coli and rare cases of streptococcus have also been associated with mastitis (Lawrence, 1989). Mastitis is usually found unilaterally; but in the rare occurrence when streptococcus is involved, it may be found bilaterally (Riordan & Auerbach, 1993). Because the site of the infection is extraductal, continued breastfeeding is recommended.

TREATMENT

Mastitis is an infection of the breast tissue, not the breast milk, so the breastfeeding relationship should not be interrupted. The infant may be reluctant to nurse on the affected side because of elevated sodium content of mastitic milk causing the breastmilk to have a salty taste (Conner, 1979). Encourage the mother to express her breastmilk if the infant refuses to breastfeed. The upper, outer quadrant of the breast has been anecdotally reported to be the most frequent site for infection to occur. Simultaneous infection in both breasts is rare, but can happen.

Recommended treatment measures for mastitis are complete emptying of the breasts, preferably by the infant; bed rest; maintenance of adequate hydration in the mother; and gentle breast massage, with application of moist heat prior to breastfeeding and ice afterwards. Applying heat increases circulation and lymph flow. Applying ice reduces inflammation. Antibiotic therapy is definitely indicated where the causative factor is bacterial in origin (Thomsen, Espersen, Maigaard, et al., 1984). Antibiotic drug choices are semisynthetic penicillins.

The usual antibiotic treatment for mastitis is a penicillinase-resistant penicillin or a cephalosporin (Riordan & Auerbach, 1993; Thomsen, Espersen, Maigaard, et al., 1985). Dicloxacillin is used as the most specific treatment of mastitis (Riordan & Auerbach, 1993). Ampicillin is not recommended due to certain staphylococci strains developing resistance to it (Fleiss, 1980; Riordan & Nichols, 1990). Analgesics may be required as a comfort measure.

Recurrent mastitis is usually the result of inadequate treatment of the initial mastitis occurrence or of delayed treatment. The breastfeeding mother must be instructed to comply with all measures of aggressive treatment to avoid recurrent mastitis.

Invasion of a fungus, such as *Candida albicans,* is a secondary complication of recurrent mastitis that is sometimes seen with postantibiotic therapy. If this occurs, the mother and infant must then be treated for the fungal infection. Alert the mother to the signs and symptoms of candidiasis and other fungal infections.

MANAGEMENT SUGGESTIONS FOR MASTITIS

Counseling strategies for the treatment of mastitis include:

1. Continue frequent breastfeeding to ensure adequate emptying of the breasts. Recommend nursing on the affected breast twice during a feeding, using different positions to thoroughly empty the breast. Begin the feeding on the unaffected side as a comfort measure; immediately switch to the affected side upon noticing the milk-ejection reflex.

2. Be sure to empty the affected breast by breastfeeding or pumping. If a breast pump is indicated, an electric-piston breast pump may be more effective in this situation. The mother should pump as often as needed to keep the breast well drained.

3. Apply warm, moist compresses to the breasts prior to a nursing session unless severely engorged. Apply ice following the session (Neville & Neifert, 1983).

4. Bed rest for the mother is strongly encouraged. Suggest that the mother take her infant to bed with her for on-demand, frequent nursings.

5. Good handwashing techniques by the mother and those assisting her with breastfeeding is encouraged.

6. Assist the mother in determining the possible cause or causes of the infection, so possible further infections may be prevented. Recurrent mastitis is usually associated with delayed or inadequate treatment of the initial infection (Lawrence, 1989).

7. Maintain adequate hydration in the mother—an elevated temperature will increase her fluid needs.

8. If symptoms do not subside within 24 hours with rest, fluids, and frequent emptying of the affected breast, contact the mother's physician for treatment by antibiotic therapy. The mother should complete her round of

treatment by antibiotics as ordered by the physician, even though her symptoms may subside sooner. Antibiotic treatment for a minimum of 10 days is usually indicated or else the mother may experience a recurrence. Medications commonly used to treat mastitis include dicloxacillin, cloxacillin, oxacillin, cephalexin, cephradine, and cefaclor. Most of these medications are taken orally, at dosage levels of 250 mg to 500 mg every six hours.

Abscessed Breast

SIGNS AND SYMPTOMS

If the breastfeeding mother continues to complain of flulike symptoms accompanied by fever and the infection site on the breast appears red, swollen, and is extremely tender to the touch, suspect a breast abscess.

CAUSATIVE FACTORS

An abscess can form from an infection if treatment is inadequate or delayed. It presents as a pus-filled area that does not respond to typical home-treatment measures.

TREATMENT

An abscess can be dangerous, and the breastfeeding mother should see her physician immediately for further diagnosis and treatment. A true abscess requires surgical drainage and antibiotic therapy. Whether the breastfeeding relationship can continue during the abscess depends on placement of the surgical drainage tube and pain associated with the abscessed area. Breastfeeding is permitted because the breastmilk is safe unless the abscess has ruptured into the ductile system (Lawrence, 1994). If for some reason breastfeeding cannot continue during the time of treatment, frequent emptying of the breasts should continue in order to maintain an adequate milk supply until the breastfeeding relationship can be reestablished. Healing sufficient to allow breastfeeding to be reestablished usually occurs within four days (Lawrence, 1994).

MANAGEMENT SUGGESTIONS FOR BREAST ABSCESS

Appropriate management of a patient with a breast abscess includes the following:

1. Contact a physician immediately for diagnosis and treatment.
2. An abscess is treated by surgical drainage and antibiotic therapy, but should also include frequent emptying of the breasts; warm, moist compresses; and bed rest.
3. If for any reason the breastfeeding relationship cannot continue during treatment, the mother should continue to express her breastmilk to help maintain her milk supply.
4. Offer increased support and encouragement to the mother.

Galactocele

SIGNS AND SYMPTOMS

A galactocele is an enclosed sac containing substances ranging from milk to a thick or oily substance that is caused by the occlusion of a milk duct. The occurrence of a galactocele is relatively uncommon. When it does develop, it tends to appear in the lactating breast. It usually palpates as a tender breast lump, but disappears at a rapid rate. If a galactocele is suspected, physician referral is indicated for further diagnosis and treatment measures.

TREATMENT

Treatment of a galactocele ranges from aspiration of the fluid-filled cyst to complete surgical removal. Breastfeeding can continue throughout the treatment phase (Lawrence, 1994).

MANAGEMENT SUGGESTIONS FOR A GALACTOCELE

Counsel the mother with a suspected galactocele to do the following:

1. Contact a physician for diagnosis and treatment.
2. Continue the breastfeeding relationship throughout the treatment phase.

Overactive Milk-Ejection Reflex

SIGNS AND SYMPTOMS

The milk-ejection reflex (MER) is a term indicating the movement of breastmilk from the alveoli, through the lactiferous ducts, to the lactiferous sinuses. As the infant sucks and nerve receptors send messages to the brain, oxytocin is released from the posterior pituitary gland and milk is ejected through the multiple openings of the nipple. An overactive MER is when the milk flow from the breast is either too fast or strong or too much for the infant to deal with (Andrusiak & Larose-Kuzenko, 1987).

CAUSATIVE FACTORS

Although to some, an overactive MER is not considered a problem, it is a problem to the mother experiencing it. The mother may present with complaints of many of the following: an infant pulling off the nipple during a breastfeeding session and crying; an infant who seems to choke easily as the reflex occurs; an infant who has increased flatus; a noise that resembles water hitting the bottom of a well or milk hitting the bottom of the nursing infant's stomach as the infant sucks and swallows; excessive leaking between and/or during a nursing session; or a milk-ejection reflex that is considered painful (Andrusiak & Larose-Kuzenko, 1987). The infant may complete feeding in less than 10 minutes per breast and may present with excessive flatus or frequent green-colored loose stools. The infant may also spit up frequently (Woolridge & Fisher, 1988).

TREATMENT

The mother with an overactive milk-ejection reflex needs continued support, encouragement, and reassurance during the temporary period while the milk-ejection reflex appears to be more than the infant can handle, so that the nursing relationship will continue. Many management suggestions should be offered to help both mother and infant cope.

MANAGEMENT SUGGESTIONS FOR AN OVERACTIVE MILK-EJECTION REFLEX

Recommend the following to the mother with an overactive milk-ejection reflex:

1. Continue frequent nursings. Although the mother may want to limit breastfeeding, encourage her to nurse frequently—this will decrease the amount of pooled milk stored in the lactiferous sinuses and may lessen

the ejection of milk flow. Encourage her to breastfeed the infant prior to crying and excessive hunger (Andrusiak & Larose-Kuzenko, 1987).

2. Nurse from one breast, instead of both, during a nursing session (Andrusiak & Larose-Kuzenko, 1987; Woolridge, Ingram, & Baum, 1990). This will decrease stimulation and may decrease the infant's frustration at the breast. The infant will continue to be well nourished while nursing from one side, receiving adequate volume, calories, and fat from the hindmilk, after feeding long enough at the first breast (Woolridge, Ingram, & Baum, 1990). If the infant awakens shortly after a nursing session, continue the nursing session on the same side, the least full breast (Riordan & Auerbach, 1993).

3. Burp the infant frequently (Andrusiak & Larose-Kuzenko, 1987).

4. Vary the breastfeeding positions used. Positions that place the infant superior to the breast may assist in controlling the milk flow (Andrusiak & Larose-Kuzenko, 1987). Encourage positioning that allows the breast-milk to pool in the infant's mouth, if needed to assist him or her in coping with the intense flow. Positions that allow the infant to remain on his side during the nursing session also work well.

5. Reassure the mother that this situation is temporary.

Impaired Milk-Ejection Reflex

SIGNS AND SYMPTOMS

Indicators of a functioning milk-ejection reflex include uterine cramping; the feeling of pins and needles in the breasts; milk leaking from the breasts; changes in the infant suck–swallow pattern after a few minutes of feeding; infant output of at least six wet disposable diapers of light-colored urine (more if cloth diapers are used) and two or more stools in 24 hours; or mother experiencing a relaxed, calm feeling (Lauwers & Woessner, 1990). The nursing mother may note all of these, but some mothers never "feel" their MER. The fact that this is considered normal should be reinforced to the nursing mother because she may believe she does not have a milk-ejection reflex if she does not feel it.

The most reliable indicators that the milk-ejection reflex has occurred are changes in the infant's sucking patterns, from rapid sucking of approximately two to three sucks per second to a deep, drawn-out sucking pattern with regular, audible swallowing. Adequate weight gain and output are also important indicators of a functioning milk-ejection reflex (Shrago & Bocar, 1990).

Mothers with an impaired milk-ejection reflex may present with complaints of an infant that does not display a long, drawn-out suck–swallow pattern. The infant may pull back from the breast after a period of nursing in frustration and dissatisfaction. He or she may not gain weight and may have less than six wet diapers in 24 hours of dark, concentrated urine.

CAUSATIVE FACTORS

The following are possible causes of an impaired MER:

1. Weak or ineffective stimulation of the nipple (McNeilly & McNeilly, 1978).
2. Factors or situations that cause the release of epinephrine or norepinephrine, which inhibit the release of oxytocin. Stress, anxiety, pain, and embarrassment are all states in which epinephrine or norepinephrine may be released (Newton & Newton, 1948).
3. History of breast surgery or breast trauma (Neifert, 1992).
4. Excessive or large amounts of alcohol intake by the nursing mother can also contribute to an impaired milk-ejection reflex (Lawrence, 1994). Amounts of ethanol that have been found to negatively affect the milk-ejection reflex measure at 1 to 2 gms per kg of maternal body weight (Cobo, 1973).

MANAGEMENT SUGGESTIONS FOR AN IMPAIRED MILK-EJECTION REFLEX

Suggest the following to the mother with an impaired milk-ejection reflex:

1. Breastfeed in a relaxed, calm area. Ensure the breastfeeding mother's comfort. Suggest relaxing music; taking the telephone off the hook or screening calls; sitting in a nest of soft, supportive pillows; etc.

2. Stimulate the breasts prior to a breastfeeding session with warm, moist compresses, warm soaks, or a warm shower; breast massage; and nipple stimulation by hand or pump.

3. Allow the infant to breastfeed for an unlimited amount of time on each breast.

4. Offer increased emotional support and encouragement. Boost the mother's confidence—worrying may only worsen the problem.

5. Educate the breastfeeding mother who is drinking alcohol on the effects of maternal alcohol intake on milk ejection.

6. Teach the mother the signs of a functioning milk-ejection reflex.

7. Teach the breastfeeding mother to watch for:
   - Audible swallowing as the infant breastfeeds.
   - At least six (disposable) to eight (cloth) wet diapers per 24 hours of light-colored urine.
   - At least two to three yellow, seedy, loose stools typical of a breastfed infant per 24 hours.
   - Adequate weight gain.

Inadequate Milk Supply

CAUSATIVE FACTORS

A mother's milk supply may depend on the amount of infant demand and intake, or the frequency and duration upon which breastfeeding takes place. The breast-feeding mother who is experiencing a low milk supply or feels the need to increase her own supply for other reasons may increase her supply at any time during the breastfeeding relationship. The breastfeeding mother's success at building her milk supply depends largely on her determination, patience, and willingness to pre-serve, as well as the infant's willingness to breastfeed. Other considerations include the health status of the mother and/or infant and whether her milk supply was established prior to the noted decrease in milk volume. The following are some of the factors that may contribute to an inadequate milk supply:

- Skipped or missed breastfeedings
- Short and infrequent breastfeedings
- Supplemental (replaced) feedings
- Complementary (added) feedings
- Beginning solids too soon
- One-sided nursing
- Mother trying to maintain a nursing schedule instead of nursing on demand
- Mother experiencing increased stress
- Mother taking birth control pills
- Poorly nourished mother (inadequate caloric intake)
- Mother unable to actively breastfeed her infant due to separation beyond her control (infant in neonatal intensive care unit)
- Menstruation
- Heavy smoking

See Module 4, *The Management of Breastfeeding,* Chapter 2, for discussion of mater-nal milk insufficiency in cases of infants with failure to thrive (FTT) or growth deficit. See Module 3, *The Science of Breastfeeding,* Chapter 2, for discussion of fac-tors that negatively influence the maternal milk volume.

MANAGEMENT SUGGESTIONS FOR AN INADEQUATE MILK SUPPLY

Recommend the following for the mother with an inadequate milk supply.

1. Breastfeed on demand, at least every two hours for an unrestricted length of time. Do not put the infant on a feeding schedule. Observe feedings for evidence of milk transfer and proper latch.
2. If for any reason the mother is unable to actively nurse the infant, she should use a breast pump to provide stimulation and milk removal. Dis-

cuss the methods and instructions for milk expression that are available and appropriate for her situation. Instructions for storage and transportation of expressed breast milk should also be discussed.

3. Breastfeed from both breasts at each feeding, allowing the infant to come off the first breast on his or her own.

4. Encourage proper nutrition and sufficient fluid intake.

5. If supplemental or complementary feedings are indicated, breastfeed first before offering, and consider alternative feeding methods for the additional feeds. Gradually decrease the amount of supplement offered as the maternal milk supply increases. Work closely with the mother during this transition period.

6. Discuss alternative birth-control methods other than the birth-control pill. Refer the client to a physician. See Module 4, *The Management of Breastfeeding*, Chapter 2, for information on contraceptive use during lactation.

7. Encourage rest and relaxation.

8. If the infant is not waking for night feedings, encourage the mother to introduce them.

POST-TEST

For questions 1 to 5, choose the best answer.

1. Candidiasis is
   A. caused by a genus of fungus called *Candida*.
   B. an infection with *Candida albicans* as the most common etiologic agent.
   C. an infection of the skin or mucous membranes.
   D. Both A and C.
   E. All of the above.

2. Signs and symptoms of candidiasis in the mother include
   A. the mother's sexual partner presenting with a rash in the groin area.
   B. pains deep in the breast that radiate upward from the nipples during or between feedings.
   C. blanched nipple tips at the end of a feeding.
   D. Both B and C.
   E. Both A and B.

3. Acute pseudomembranous candidiasis in the breastfed infant
   A. is always visually obvious when the mother is also exhibiting signs and symptoms of candidiasis.
   B. is one of the most common forms of oral candidiasis.
   C. may appear on the perianal area, throat, and oral cavity.
   D. Both B and C.
   E. All of the above.

4. Trauma, vascular engorgement, or a carcinoma may all cause a nipple discharge that appears
   A. purulent.
   B. bloody.
   C. multicolored and sticky.
   D. green.

5. _____ is a bilaterally occurring, extreme, inappropriate, or continued leaking of a milky discharge in women of childbearing age.
   A. Lactation
   B. Leaking
   C. Galactorrhea
   D. Galactocele

For questions 6 to 12, choose the best answer from the following key:
A. True   B. False

6. The fungus *Candida* may be easily transferred between the mother and infant. It may also be transferred among family members if hygiene is poor.

7. A mother with herpes simplex virus should wean her infant from the breast immediately upon diagnosis.

8. The breastfeeding mother's sexual partner should not kiss her breast during an outbreak of herpes simplex virus.

9. When the breastfeeding mother wears breast shells to help correct flat nipples, she should wear them around the clock in order to gain the greatest benefit.

10. Foods containing red and yellow dyes have been linked to reports of pink- or orange-colored breastmilk.

11. Minocycline hydrochloride, a semisynthetic derivative of tetracycline, has been found in the breastmilk of women taking this tetracycline and is associated with black milk.

12. Pathological engorgement can occur at any point during the breastfeeding relationship when the breasts are not emptied and milk accumulation is prolonged.

For questions 13 to 16, choose the best answer from the following key:

    A. **Moderate-to-severe retraction**   C. **Protracting normal nipple**
    B. **Complete inversion**   D. **Inverted appearing/pseudo-inverted**

13. The nipple does not respond to manual pressure because adhesions bind the nipple inward; very rarely, there is congenital absence of the nipple.

14. Nipple moves forward; considered a normal functional response. No special interventions are needed.

15. Retracts to a level even with or behind the surrounding areola. Intervention is helpful to stretch the nipple outward and improve protractability.

16. The nipple appears inverted but moves outward to protraction with manual pressure or when cold.

For questions 17 to 20, choose the best answer from the following key:

    A. **if responses 1, 2, and 3 are correct**   C. **if responses 2 and 4 are correct**
    B. **if responses 1 and 3 are correct**   D. **if all responses are correct**

17. Plugged duct symptoms may include
    1. a tender lump.
    2. a temperature above 100.4°F.
    3. redness in the area of complaint.
    4. flulike symptoms.

18. Abscessed breast symptoms may include
    1. pus-filled area.
    2. mother with flulike symptoms.
    3. fever.
    4. red and swollen breast.

19. Mastitis symptoms may include
    1. breast soreness and redness.
    2. flulike symptoms.
    3. temperature above 100.4°F.
    4. pus-filled area.

20. Pathological engorgement
    1. occurs during the first week postpartum.
    2. is characterized by hot, swollen, red, and shiny-appearing breasts.
    3. may lead to infant rejection due to salty taste of milk.
    4. occurs at any point during the breastfeeding relationship.

SECTION D

Infant-Related Problems

Jan B. Simpson, RN, BSN, IBCLC

LEARNING OBJECTIVES

At the completion of this section, the learner will be able to do the following:

1. Identify possible causes of breast refusal by the infant and provide recommendations for reinitiating and maintaining a successful breastfeeding relationship.
2. List possible causes of sucking difficulties and offer recommendations for management.
3. Discuss the possible side effects of the early introduction of artificial teats.
4. Discuss management suggestions for the infant presenting with nipple confusion.
5. Identify signs and symptoms of an infant displaying a weak suck and offer suggestions for management.
6. Recognize ankyloglossia and discuss possible treatment options, if indicated.
7. Discuss possible causes of tongue thrusting in the infant and offer recommendations for management.
8. Recognize signs of an infant presenting with a retracted or curled tongue and offer recommendations for management.
9. Discuss the characteristics displayed by an infant presenting with a tonic bite reflex and offer management suggestions.
10. Explain the possible effects of complementary and supplementary feeds in relation to milk production, milk intake, and sucking behavior of the breastfeeding infant.

OUTLINE

PRE-TEST

For questions 1 to 8, choose the best answer.

1. An infant may refuse the breast because of a change in the taste of the breast-milk, which may be caused by

    A. mastitis.
    B. malignancy.
    C. menstrual cycle.
    D. All of the above.

2. In positioning an infant at the breast, the baby should be

    A. ventral surface to ventral surface with the mother.
    B. held in the cradle hold with his or her head and body turned to the breast.
    C. positioned so that the head is always in straight alignment with the body.
    D. Both A and C.
    E. All of the above.

3. During a breastfeeding session, infants should be observed

    A. rooting and sucking.
    B. rooting, sucking, and swallowing.
    C. sucking, swallowing, and burping.
    D. None of the above.

4. The premature infant often presents with sucking difficulties due to

    A. his or her gestational age of less than 37 weeks and developmental immaturity.
    B. his or her gestational age of less than 40 weeks and small size.
    C. a delay in putting him or her to the breast.
    D. Both A and C.
    E. Both B and C.

5. Many premature infants exhibit

    A. a rapid suck that occurs when no liquid is introduced into the infant's oral cavity.
    B. a pattern of slower sucking that occurs when liquid is introduced into the infant's oral cavity.
    C. no suck, unless the infant is at least 34 weeks gestational age.
    D. a rapid suck at 34 to 36 weeks gestational age and a pattern of slower sucking at 36 weeks gestational age and older.
    E. Both C and D.

6. Infants who present with a weak suck may benefit greatly from the mother supporting her breast using the

    A. V hold.
    B. dancer hand position.
    C. C hold.
    D. breast sling.

7. Nipple confusion may lead to

    A. inefficient sucking at the breast.
    B. engorgement.
    C. plugged ducts.
    D. mastitis.
    E. All of the above.

8. Which best describes what happens as the infant sucks at the breast?
    A. When sucking from the breast, the infant's tongue is extended over the lower alveolar ridge and is pushed upward and forward to help control the flow of milk from the nipple.
    B. When sucking from the breast, the infant's tongue extends beyond the lower alveolar ridge, forming a trough and cupping the breast. The tongue remains in place over the lower alveolar ridge throughout the feeding.
    C. Removal of milk from the breast occurs by the peristaltic-like stripping movement of the tongue and the opening and closing movement of the mandible.
    D. Both A and C.
    E. Both B and C.

For questions 9 to 14, choose the best answer from the following key:

   A. **Weak suck**   C. **Tongue thrusting**
   B. **Ankyloglossia**   D. **Tonic bite reflex**

9. The breast continually falls out of the infant's mouth during a breastfeeding session.

10. The infants who most often present with this problem have a history of early introduction of artificial teats or were born prematurely or with a neurological problem.

11. Use of the dancer hand position may prove very helpful.

12. A congenital syndrome.

13. Infant bites down on anything touching the inside of the mouth.

14. Frenotomy is one of the treatments used to correct this.

For questions 15 to 20, choose the best answer from the following key:

   A. **True**   B. **False**

15. Breastmilk does not completely meet the fluid needs of infants living in warm climate areas.

16. Colostrum is a physiologic secretion and will not cause an irritating effect like a foreign substance that may be given to the infant to help detect a possible tracheoesophageal fistula. It is readily absorbed in the respiratory tree if it is aspirated.

17. Offering the breastfed infant complementary and supplementary feeds helps reduce jaundice by decreasing the bilirubin levels.

18. A breastfeeding mother's milk production is greatly affected by the introduction of additional or replacement feeds.

19. There is no reason for a breastfed infant to ever need complementary or supplementary feeds.

20. The hospital routine of offering free infant-formula gift packs to breastfeeding mothers may have a negative impact on a successful breastfeeding relationship.

Refusal of the Breast

An infant's refusal of the breast (nursing strike) can be related to a number of causes or situations. This is a frustrating time for both the mother and the infant. At times, the breastfeeding mother may misinterpret a nursing strike as the infant weaning himself or herself (Winchell, 1992). When counseling the mother who is experiencing breast refusal, determine the cause of the refusal; offer support and encouragement as well. In addition, it is extremely important to educate the mother on maintaining her milk supply.

CAUSATIVE FACTORS

Determining the cause of the breast refusal can be an extremely frustrating experience in itself. The cause may be related to the mother's health, the infant's health, breastfeeding techniques, the breastmilk itself, the developmental stage the infant is going through, or various external sources. While refusal of the breast may occur at any time during the breastfeeding relationship, it most often occurs between the ages of seven and nine months (Riordan & Auerbach, 1993). The introduction of bottles and pacifiers is the most common reason for refusal of the breast (Newman, 1990; Winchell, 1992). The following is a list of the many possible causative factors of breast refusal by an infant:

- Engorgement
- Mastitis, which may give the breast milk a salty taste
- A breast malignancy, which may give the milk a bad taste
- The menstrual cycle, which may also influence the taste and supply of milk
- An overactive milk-ejection reflex
- An inhibited milk-ejection reflex
- Increased stress or an emotional upset experienced by the mother
- Use of perfumes, deodorants, shampoos, soaps, laundry detergents, or similar products. Introduction of new products may also create a refusal.
- Spicy or other strong-flavored foods eaten by the mother, which may change the milk flavor
- Heavy smoking by the mother, which may change the milk flavor as well as the milk-ejection reflex and milk supply
- Use of nipple creams or ointments
- Poor positioning techniques
- Poor latch-on techniques
- An upset in the infant's routine
- Nipple confusion caused by early introduction of bottles or pacifiers
- Infant with an infection in one or both ears
- Infant with nasal congestion
- Infant with teething discomfort
- Infant who received a birth injury (facial trauma, hematoma, bruising, scalp laceration, shoulder dystocia)
- An easily distracted infant
- Infant with an oral candida infection

- Infant with oral herpes simplex virus (HSV) lesions
- Infant receiving oral trauma, such as frequent suctioning
- Infant with ankyloglossia

MANAGEMENT SUGGESTIONS FOR REFUSAL OF THE BREAST

Guidelines for counseling the mother whose infant is refusing the breast include:

1. Discuss measures to prevent engorgement, mastitis, and other breast-related problems. Instruct the mother to continue to offer the affected breast but, if refusal continues, expression is indicated. In the case of mastitis, the salty taste will probably subside within approximately seven days and the nursing relationship can continue.

2. Make the breastfeeding mother aware that some infants have been reported to have rejected the breasts at the beginning of the menstrual cycle, but that this is temporary. Breastmilk expression may be indicated to prevent overfullness and to maintain the milk supply until the breastfeeding is reestablished.

3. Educate the mother with an overactive milk-ejection reflex about ways to help her infant cope during the temporary period. (See the discussion on overactive milk-ejection reflex in Section C of this chapter.)

4. Educate the mother with an inhibited milk-ejection reflex (MER) about ways she can work on establishing the MER. (See the discussion on inhibited milk-ejection reflex in Section C of this chapter.)

5. Discuss things that can be done to help the breastfeeding mother reduce her stress level. Discuss relaxation techniques.

6. If the mother has had a positive breastfeeding experience prior to the refusal, question her about any recent introduction of new brands of soap, perfume, shampoo, deodorant, laundry detergent, or other similar products. She may need to discontinue using the new product while she is breastfeeding, or she may be able to change brands and reestablish the breastfeeding relationship (Lawrence, 1989).

7. Ask the mother for a 24-hour diet recall prior to the refusal. Certain foods or drinks may have changed the taste of her milk. Alcohol has also been shown to affect the flavor of breastmilk and subsequently decrease the quantity taken by the infant (Mennella & Beauchamp, 1991).

8. If the mother is a heavy smoker, discuss the possibility of decreasing the number of cigarettes smoked per day or quitting for her health, as well as for the infant. If she must smoke, encourage her not to smoke while breastfeeding, to smoke after a breastfeeding session instead of prior to, and not to smoke around the infant.

9. Encourage the mother to use her own breastmilk on her nipples. The smell or taste of some artificial creams put on the breast may be the cause of the infant's refusal.

10. Assist the mother with proper positioning and latch-on techniques. Make sure that the infant's head and body are in alignment while nursing and that the infant has a proper areolar grasp.

11. Encourage the mother not to introduce the artificial teat of a bottle until four weeks of age or later, if possible, to help prevent nipple confusion. If supplemental or complementary feeds are necessary, encourage alternative feeding methods (cup, dropper, spoon, finger feeding, nursing supplementary system). Studies have substantiated the relationship between use of supplementary bottles in the early weeks and early termination of the breastfeeding relationship (Ryan, Wysong, Martinez, et al., 1990; Samuels et al., 1990).

12. If the infant is experiencing an ear infection or congestion, breastfeeding may be uncomfortable. Encourage nursing in an upright position, such as the football hold, because this may take pressure off the ears and aid in nasal drainage. If only one ear is affected and the infant is nursing in a vertical position, avoid lying him on that ear. Feedings that are short in duration and frequent may prove beneficial.

13. An infant experiencing teething discomfort may refuse to nurse. Rubbing the gums prior to breastfeeding with a cool cloth, providing a chewing toy, or giving medication (if recommended by the infant's physician or dentist) may encourage breastfeeding. Reassure the mother that this is a temporary situation.

14. Discuss the symptoms of thrush with the breastfeeding mother. An oral candida infection may cause the nursing infant great discomfort. Physician referral is indicated for confirmed diagnosis and treatment.

15. The developmental stage the infant is going through may change the breastfeeding relationship. The infant may be more interested in the things occurring around him or her, or may be easily distracted. Encourage the mother to breastfeed in a quiet, relaxed area, free from distractions. Some mothers find nursing in a dimly lit or dark room is effective. Many infants are highly sensitive to loud voices. The mother may need to be nonvocal or speak in a low, soft manner when nursing. Encourage the mother to attempt to nurse the infant while he or she is in a light sleep.

16. A physical injury may make nursing uncomfortable for the infant. Encourage the breastfeeding mother to try various nursing positions to find one that is comfortable for the infant. Infants with shoulder dystocia or whose deliveries were accomplished by vacuum extraction or forceps may be more sensitive to positioning.

Sucking Difficulties

Proper positioning, latching-on, and sucking are necessary for an adequate intake of milk by the breastfeeding infant. The counselor and the breastfeeding mother should observe for indicators of an effective suck during a breastfeeding session. See Sections B and C in Chapter 1 of this module for information on proper positioning and how to assess feeding at the breast.

SIGNS INDICATING EFFICIENT SUCK

An efficient suck by the infant of a mother with an adequate milk volume will result in milk transfer. Signs of an efficient suck include:

1. Infant should be properly positioned and latched-on to the breast, with the ventral surface of the infant to the ventral surface of the mother and the infant's head in straight alignment with his or her body.
2. When actively breastfeeding, the infant's tongue should be extended beyond the lower alveolar ridge, forming a trough to cup the breast (Weber, Woolridge, & Baum, 1986). Removal of milk from the breast occurs by a peristaltic-like movement of the infant's tongue and the opening and closing action of the mandible (Woolridge, 1986).
3. After the milk-ejection reflex occurs, audible swallowing must be noted. Swallowing will be noted after every one to two sucks. This is the most reliable indicator of milk intake by the infant (Shrago & Bocar, 1990). Swallowing may not be audible during colostrum production.
4. The neonate should have at least six wet disposable diapers of light-colored urine and at least 2 to 3 seedy loose stools in a 24-hour period.
5. Ideally, the infant should regain his birth weight within 10 days to two weeks, continuing with an average gain of 4 to 7 ounces per week in the first month. See Module 3, *The Science of Breastfeeding*, Chapter 3, for weight gain recomendations in infancy.

POSSIBLE CAUSES OF SUCKING DIFFICULTIES

All infants should be observed rooting, sucking, and swallowing during a breastfeeding session. If abnormalities or difficulties with the process are noticed, immediate action must be taken to find the etiology and assistance given for correction. There are various conditions or circumstances that may interfere with the infant's ability to suck. Infants who are born prematurely may display an inadequate or diminished suck, depending on the infant's developmental maturity. A mother who has been medicated in labor or afterward may have an infant who is sleepy or has a lazy suck for a period of time. A successful breastfeeding relationship is possible, although these breastfeeding mothers may need additional assistance, support, and encouragement. Other conditions that may affect the infant's suck include neurological impairments, Down syndrome, neuromuscular disorders, infections of the central nervous system, cleft lip, cleft palate, macroglossia, ankyloglossia, and prematurity.

Sucking difficulty is often seen in premature infants. The premature infant, born before the completion of the thirty-seventh week of gestation and often weighing less than 2,500 gms (5 lbs., 8 oz.), may present with various problems that interfere with his ability to suck properly at the breast. There may be a delay in putting the infant to the breast because of his or her prematurity or its associated problems. If this happens and breastfeeding is delayed, the mother should be instructed on use of the electric breast pump.

When the premature infant is able to be put to the breast, he or she may present with an inadequate suck, e.g., tongue thrusting, nipple confusion, or a weak suck. The mother of a premature infant can breastfeed and should be strongly encouraged to do so. She will require additional breastfeeding assistance, support, and encouragement to help overcome the obstacles she may encounter. See Module 4, *The Management of Breastfeeding*, Chapter 3, for more on breastfeeding the premature infant.

Many premature infants have the ability to exhibit a nonnutritive suck, a rapid suck that occurs when no liquid is introduced into the infant's oral cavity, but do not have the coordination required to have a nutritive suck, a pattern of slower sucking that occurs when liquid is introduced into the infant's oral cavity. These infants will experience feeding difficulties and may benefit greatly from various feeding methods as transitional measures to sucking at the breast, such as finger feeding.

The mother putting her premature infant to the breast will need to be aware that he or she will tire easily and may have to be awakened for the feeding. The baby's rooting reflex, along with sucking capabilities, will be weakened; and he or she will need assistance with getting the nipple in the mouth, keeping it there, and maintaining suction. Infants presenting with a weak suck may benefit greatly from the mother supporting her breast using the dancer hand position, because otherwise the weight of the breast may pull the nipple from the infant's mouth. This hold allows the mother to support the weight of her breast and support her infant's jaw and chin during the feeding. This support may help keep the infant from tiring so easily at the breast and allow the infant to use all his or her energy for breastfeeding.

Another commonly seen cause of sucking difficulties is the early introduction of artificial teats (bottle nipples, pacifiers, nipple shields). For the breastfeeding infant, introduction of artificial teats may begin a process of inadequate sucking at the breast or even total refusal of the breast. This can lead to numerous health problems for both mother and infant. The most common problem, nipple confusion, occurs because of the different sucking actions required for the breast and bottle. When sucking from an artificial teat, the infant only opens his or her mouth a small amount and the lips close around the small rubber teat. The infant's tongue is pushed forward but does not trough the nipple as in breastfeeding (Ardan, 1958). Little if any jaw action is required while sucking from a bottle.

When sucking from the breast, the infant's mouth is open wide, as when yawning, and the lips are flanged and form a seal around the areola area because a large portion of the breast is taken into the mouth. The infant's tongue extends beyond the lower alveolar ridge, forming a trough and cupping the breast (Weber, Woolridge, & Baum, 1986). The removal of milk from the mother's breast occurs by a peristaltic-like movement of the infant's tongue and the opening and closing action of the mandible (Woolridge, 1986). These combined movements act together to express milk from the lactiferous sinuses of the breast to the back of the infant's oral cavity. As the mandible is opened, the lactiferous sinuses refill (Woolridge, 1986).

With the early introduction of artificial teats, nipple confusion may easily develop. Nipple confusion occurs when the infant attempts to suck the breast as he would suck a bottle (Minchin, 1985). It causes an inefficient suck at the breast, which can lead to inadequate milk intake, engorgement, plugged ducts, mastitis, inadequate milk production, and sore nipples, which may lead to untimely weaning from the breast.

Poor hospital routines may initially subject the breastfeeding mother and infant to sucking difficulties by the early introduction of unnecessary artificial teats, in the form of pacifiers, nipple shields, or bottle teats. Supplementary or complementary feeds are not necessary unless medically indicated and ordered by the physician. The infant may become nipple-confused and be satisfied by the formula or water and refuse the breast or spend insufficient time at the breast. The relationship between supplementary bottles offered to a breastfed infant and early weaning has been well documented (Ryan, Wysong, Martinez et al., 1990; Samuels, Margen, Schoen, et al., 1985). If additional feeds are medically indicated, feeding methods other than the artificial teat are encouraged (supplemental nursing systems, dropper, spoon, cup, finger feeding, periodontal syringe).

Excessive use of pacifiers may lead to multiple problems, such as slow weight gain, engorgement, inadequate milk supply, because less time is spent at the breast since the infant's sucking needs are being met by the pacifier. The structure of the pacifier, as well as the nipple shield and bottle teat, differs from the breast, and the infant's sucking action at the breast may become ineffective. Pacifiers should not be used to replace frequent breastfeeding.

Nipple shields should only be used as a last resort, and the mother should be instructed on proper use if they must be used. Nipple shields may not only cause nipple confusion, but may also decrease the amount of milk intake the infant receives, possibly leading to engorgement from inadequate emptying of the breasts and to an inadequate milk supply (Auerbach, 1990; Frantz, 1982).

Nipple Confusion

Introducing artificial teats to the breastfeeding infant may begin a process of inadequate sucking at the breast or even total refusal of the breast, which can lead to numerous health problems for both the breastfeeding mother and infant. The most common problem is called nipple confusion; it develops because, as described in the previous section, the action of the mouth, tongue, and mandible differs from breast to bottle (Minchin, 1985).

With the early or frequent introduction of artificial teats, nipple confusion may easily develop. It often leads to an inefficient suck at the breast, which can lead to many problems (inadequate milk intake, engorgement, plugged ducts, mastitis, inadequate milk production, and sore nipples), which may lead to untimely weaning from the breast.

To evaluate whether daily bottle use negatively impacts on breastfeeding, Cronewett and associates (1992) enrolled 121 women in a study and randomly assigned them to either a group who would offer one bottle a day to their infants between two and six weeks or who would breastfeed exclusively. In practice, the bottle group gave an average of five to nine bottles per week, the exclusively breastfeeding group were allowed to give up to two bottles per week, and almost all received at least two bottles in the first week. Mothers who reported severe problems had infants more likely to receive bottles in the hospital. At 12-weeks postpartum, 93% of the exclusive group were still breastfeeding, compared to 83% of the planned bottle group. Almost one-third of the mothers whose babies received bottles in the hospital reported severe breastfeeding problems, while only 14% of the mothers who did not receive (excessive) bottles experienced severe problems. The authors minimize these differences in their discussion, but further data is needed to determine how much stronger the differences would be if truly no interference in breastfeeding occurs, as originally planned in this study.

MANAGEMENT SUGGESTIONS FOR THE INFANT WITH NIPPLE CONFUSION

Maher (1988) provides the following management suggestions for the infant experiencing nipple confusion:

1. *Day One:* Offer the infant experiencing nipple confusion supplementary feeds, preferably breastmilk, using methods other than the bottle. Do not attempt breastfeeding at this time.

2. *Day Two:* Continue to offer supplemental feedings as suggested above. When possible, have the mother feed near her bare breast. Offer the breast prior to and in between feeds. Do not force the infant to take the breast if he or she is uninterested.

3. After the infant begins taking the breast as mentioned above, begin putting him or her to the breast prior to his probable time of next being hungry. Encourage skin-to-skin contact while breastfeeding, if possible. If the infant continues to refuse the breast, continue instructions of day two.

4. The infant will usually begin breastfeeding at this point. The mother should be instructed on ways to tell if the infant is being adequately nourished. Weight gain should be monitored carefully. See Module 4, *The Management of Breastfeeding*, Chapter 2, for information on management strategies for growth deficit.

5. Avoid artificial nipples for several weeks to prevent a repeat of nipple confusion and to allow the infant time to learn to breastfeed.

Weak Suck

SIGNS AND SYMPTOMS

Signs that may show that an infant is experiencing problems due to a weak suck include: the breast continually falling out of the infant's mouth during a breast-feeding session, especially if it happens when the mother moves even the slightest amount during the feeding; milk leaking from the infant's mouth while nursing; or the infant easily choking on the breastmilk while breastfeeding (Maher, 1988). Early introduction of artificial teats, poor muscle tone, neurological impairment, immature nervous system, sickness, and weakness from inadequate nourishment may cause an infant to have a weak suck. Identification of the infant with a weak suck should be made as soon as possible, and corrective actions begun before the mother's milk supply diminishes. Physician referral is indicated.

The mother of an infant with a weak suck may experience problems due to the decreased breast stimulation. She may initially experience engorgement, then a decreased milk supply due to the lack of stimulation and the small amount of milk being taken from the breast. It may be necessary for the mother to supplement breastfeeding, preferably with her own expressed breastmilk (hindmilk), in order to assure that the infant receives his or her caloric demands and nourishment needs. Advise the mother to avoid using artificial teats for this supplementation and to consider alternative feeding methods, such as a supplemental nursing system, dropper, spoon, cup, or finger feeding. Simultaneously, the mother should work at increasing her own milk supply.

The breastfeeding mother should be taught to observe for effective sucking. She should be instructed to listen for audible swallowing while her infant is at the breast. The newborn should have at least six wet disposable diapers (more if cloth) of light-colored urine and at least two to three stools within a 24-hour period. A weight gain of four to seven ounces per week is desired before decreasing and omitting the supplemental feeds (Maher, 1988).

MANAGEMENT SUGGESTIONS FOR INFANT WITH A WEAK SUCK

Suggest the following strategies for the infant with a weak suck:

1. Physician referral is indicated. Have the mother make an appointment for a physical for the infant to rule out any type of physical problem that could be causing the weak suck. The infant will require ongoing medical evaluation and supervision during this time.

2. Have the mother try several nursing positions to see if sucking improves. Infants that have poor muscle tone will many times suck better in the lying down or cradle hold positions.

3. Prior to breastfeeding, stimulate the infant's lips by circling around them with a finger. Repeat this technique three times clockwise and three times counterclockwise. This may assist the infant in obtaining a better seal on the breast.

4. Assure proper positioning and latching-on.

5. Use the dancer hand position to support the breast and infant's jaw and chin while breastfeeding.

6. Encourage short, frequent breastfeeding sessions—at least every two hours during the day hours and at least one session during the night.

7. Encourage measures that will assist the mother in maintaining and increasing her milk supply, such as use of the breast pump.

8. The infant with a weak suck may temporarily need supplementation to ensure adequate nutritional and caloric intake. This may be gradually decreased as weight gain begins, with an average gain of four to seven ounces per week, and medical approval from the infant's physician.

9. The infant should have at least six wet disposable diapers (more if cloth) of light-colored urine and at least two to three stools within a 24-hour time frame during the newborn period.

10. Offer increased support and encouragement to the mother.

Ankyloglossia

SIGNS AND SYMPTOMS

Ankyloglossia (also referred to as tongue-tied, short frenulum, or tight frenulum) is a congenital syndrome that is characterized by the lingual frenulum (tissue that attaches the tongue to the floor of the mouth) presenting to be too short, too tight, or attached at the tip of the tongue, which causes the tongue tip to appear heart-shaped. Ankyloglossia is hereditary, and upon careful research or interview, the mother, father, or another close relative of the infant may also have ankyloglossia. Ankyloglossia may or may not restrict the tongue movement. If it does, breastfeeding difficulties may arise soon after birth (Marmet, Shell, & Marmet, 1990; Notestine, 1990). Impaired action of the tongue may negatively affect the breastfeeding relationship. A significant component in the effective removal of milk from the mother's breast is the tongue's mobility (Hazelbaker, 1993; Woolridge, 1986). Appropriate peristalsis of the tongue may be hindered by a tight lingual frenulum (Marmet, Shell, & Marmet, 1990).

The nursing mother may present with chief complaints of severe nipple pain from the inappropriate sucking behavior presented by the infant. The nipple pain may be caused by the infant biting down on the areolar tissue with his gums to hold the breast since his tongue cannot reach or maintain a position on the lower alveolar ridge or lip. Trauma may arise from the infant's attempted sucking because of friction on the nipples as the tongue is snapped back to the floor of the oral cavity by the tight frenulum. The role of the tongue in the sucking process is crucial: This condition may lead to poor infant weight gain caused by inadequate sucking at the breast, inadequate emptying of the breast, mastitis, and inadequate milk production and supply (Hazelbaker, 1993; Marmet, Shell, & Marmet, 1990).

ASSESSMENT OF ANKYLOGLOSSIA

Until the recent publication of Hazelbaker's (1993) thesis on ankyloglossia, the assessment of ankyloglossia was left to the individual's visual assessment and choice of criteria. There had not been a uniform or systematic approach to determine the degree of ankyloglossia or need for treatment. Some health-care providers used the criteria of a visual assessment of a heart-shaped tongue, while others used the inability of the infant to protrude the tongue over the lower lip, sounds produced while attempting to suck at the breast, or just whether the tongue seems to lack normal mobility. Hazelbaker developed an Assessment Tool for Lingual Frenulum Function (ATLFF). She describes ATLFF as a primary step toward providing data that is required to make determinations on the impact of ankyloglossia on the tongue's function as related to breastfeeding. See Table 2D–1 for a description of the ATLFF.

SURGICAL TREATMENT OF ANKYLOGLOSSIA

Treatment of ankyloglossia is somewhat controversial, and parents of an infant with ankyloglossia may find it difficult to locate someone willing to perform the

Table 2D–1   The Assessment Tool for Lingual Frenulum

Function Items	Appearance Items

LATERALIZATION

2 Complete
1 Body of tongue but not tongue tip
0 None

LIFT OF TONGUE

2 Tip to midmouth
1 Only edges to midmouth
0 Tip stays at lower alveolar ridge *or* tip rises to midmouth only with jaw closure

EXTENSION OF TONGUE

2 Tip over lower lip
1 Tip over lower gum only
0 Neither of the above *or* anterior or midtongue humps

SPREAD OF ANTERIOR TONGUE

2 Complete
1 Moderate *or* partial
0 Little *or* none

CUPPING

2 Entire edge, firm cup
1 Side edges only, moderate cup
0 Poor *or* no cup

  14 = Perfect score (regardless of Appearance item score).
  11 = Acceptable if Appearance item score is 10.
<11 = Function impaired. Frenotomy should be consid-
      ered if management fails.
Frenotomy necessary if Appearance item score is <8.

APPEARANCE OF TONGUE WHEN LIFTED

2 Round *or* square
1 Slight cleft in tip apparent
0 Heart-shaped

ELASTICITY OF FRENULUM

2 Very elastic (excellent)
1 Moderately elastic
0 Little *or* no elasticity

**LENGTH OF LINGUAL FRENULUM WHEN
TONGUE LIFTED**

2 More than 1 cm
1 1 cm
0 Less than 1 cm

**ATTACHMENT OF LINGUAL FRENULUM
TO TONGUE**

2 Posterior to tip
1 At tip
0 Notched tip

**ATTACHMENT OF LINGUAL FRENULUM TO
INFERIOR ALVEOLAR RIDGE**

2 Attached to floor of mouth *or* well below ridge
1 Attached just below ridge
0 Attached at ridge

  10 = Perfect score if Function item score is higher than 11.
   8 = Acceptable score if Function item score is higher
      than 11.
<8 = Acceptable score only if Function item score is 14.
Frenotomy recommended if Function item score is <14.

Source: Hazelbaker, AK (1993). *The Assessment Tool for Lingual Frenulum Function (ATLFF): Use in a Lactation Consultant Private Practice.* Self-published. Reprinted with permission. (For more information regarding the ATLFF, contact Alison K. Hazelbaker, 5095 Olentangy River Rd., Columbus OH 43235.)

simple procedure to help correct the problem. Some medical practitioners do not agree with the surgical procedure to correct ankyloglossia, stating that it has no functional significance and that as the child grows, the frenulum will stretch or tear on its own. Ankyloglossia can cause breastfeeding problems and lactation consultants must educate pediatric surgeons about the effects of ankyloglossia on breastfeeding.

Dentists have recognized that the surgical reduction of the abnormal lingual frenum is indicated if it interferes with the infant's nursing. Because this is a surgical procedure, trained medical professionals must perform the procedure to prevent injury to tongue muscles, infection, and increased bleeding. A thorough knowledge of the anatomy of the mouth is critical. Physicians; dentists; oral surgeons; ears, nose, and throat specialists; and general or pediatric surgeons may perform this surgical treatment.

A frenotomy is one of the surgical techniques used to correct ankyloglossia in the infant. It is a simple procedure and may be done on an outpatient basis in the doctor's office (Hazelbaker, 1993). No anesthetic, medication, or stitching of the area is required, because the frenulum is poorly vascularized and poorly supplied with nerves. The infant feels little pain and experiences little if any bleeding at all. The doctor clips or makes an incision in the frenulum with sterile scissors which allows for free movement of the tongue. The infant is immediately put to the breast to feed. Many mothers report immediate improvement of the infant's suck and decreased nipple discomfort, while a few mothers report having to assist the infant in retraining his or her suck (Notestine, 1990).

Two other surgical procedures are used to treat ankyloglossia. Stripping the frenulum with a sharp instrument is usually done following an incision of the frenulum. This procedure is dangerous because of the damage it does to the underlying structures of the tongue. A frenectomy, an excision of the lingual frenulum, usually requires hospitalization and anesthesia because it is a more extensive procedure (Hazelbaker, 1993; Notestine, 1990).

MANAGEMENT SUGGESTIONS FOR ANKYLOGLOSSIA

Suggest the following for the infant with ankyloglossia:

1. Use ATLFF to determine whether ankyloglossia is the main cause of a breastfeeding problem.
2. Encourage the parents to discuss the possibilities of clipping the frenulum, including the benefits and risks, with a trained medical professional, such as a physician or dentist.

Tongue Thrusting

SIGNS AND SYMPTOMS

The breastfeeding mother may present with chief complaints of the nursing infant being unable to latch on to the breast or suck efficiently because of the thrusting of the infant's tongue. By pushing the tongue forward, the infant pushes or spits the nipple from his or her mouth. The mother may complain of nipple soreness on the tips of her nipples.

Infants most often presenting with this problem have a history of early introduction of artificial teats, which resulted in nipple confusion, or were born either prematurely or with a neurological problem (Maher, 1988). The breastfeeding mother should be carefully interviewed about the infant's medical history in order to assist in discovering etiologies and corrective measures for the tongue thrusting.

MANAGEMENT SUGGESTIONS FOR TONGUE THRUSTING

Suggest the following for the infant with tongue thrust:

1. Ensure proper positioning and latching-on of the infant at breast.
2. Instruct the mother to try nursing the infant while he or she is swaddled (Maher, 1988).
3. Instruct the mother to try nursing the infant with his or her chin pointed downward, almost touching the infant's chest (Maher, 1988).
4. If the infant continues to push the breast from his or her mouth, instruct the mother on using the following technique, referred to as "walking back on the tongue" (Maher, 1988, p. 12):
   A. Gently stroke the infant's cheek in the direction towards his mouth, brushing his lips a few times.
   B. Use a clean index finger with a well-trimmed nail and massage the outside of the infant's gums. Begin in the midline of the gum and move toward the sides of the gum.
   C. As the infant's mouth opens, press down firmly on the tongue tip with the tip of the index finger and count 1–2–3.
   D. Release the pressure, and move back on the tongue repeating this one or two more times. Avoid gagging the infant.
   E. Repeat this procedure 3 or 4 times prior to each breastfeeding session.
5. Discuss management suggestions for nipple confusion.

Retracted Tongue or Tip of Tongue Curls

SIGNS AND SYMPTOMS

If the breastfeeding mother is unable to observe the breastfeeding infant's tongue extended beyond the lower alveolar ridge while feeding and is complaining of nipple soreness to the sides of her nipple or possibly the nipple tip, she may be experiencing an infant whose tongue is retracted. The tongue tip tends to rub the sides of the nipple, or sometimes the end, producing tenderness and trauma because of the retraction.

If the mother complains of soreness and a vertical red stripe is noted across the end of the nipple, it may be due to a tongue that curls up. Often, when the tongue curls up, the frenulum may rub against the nipple. She may report noting a clicking or smacking sound during feedings. This is caused by the continued loss of suction. The infant may be gaining weight slowly, and audible swallowing is rarely noted during a feeding.

MANAGEMENT SUGGESTIONS FOR THE INFANT WITH A RETRACTED OR CURLED TONGUE

Suggest the following strategies when an infant retracts or curls his or her tongue during feedings:

1. Swaddle the infant while nursing and position the infant with his or her chin pointing downward, almost touching the chest. This may help the tongue to relax and stay down (Maher, 1988).

2. Encourage nursing in a position that requires the infant to sit up. This promotes alertness and assists the tongue to perform properly.

3. If no improvement is noted after trying the above suggestions, the mother may try the following finger exercise: Hold the infant face down and support him or her on the mother's forearm. Support the infant's forehead with the palm of the hand. Offer him or her a clean finger to suck on (padded side of finger against the infant's palate, nail side down). Suggest the mother walk around with the infant in this position for no longer than five minutes. If the infant continues to refuse to suck on the finger, and the mother's nipple soreness does not improve, begin suck training techniques with the infant.

4. Monitor infant weight gain carefully. If weight gain is poor, see Module 4, *The Management of Breastfeeding*, Chapter 2, for information on managing growth deficit.

Tonic Bite Reflex

SIGNS AND SYMPTOMS

An infant born with a tonic bite reflex consistently bites down on anything touching the inside of his mouth. This reflex may only be present for a few days or may continue for a longer period of time. The mother may present with complaints of sore nipples that turn white by the end of a nursing session caused by the infant biting down on the nipple. If management suggestions do not improve the situation or weight loss occurs, the mother may need to express her breastmilk and feed the infant using alternative methods until the clenching begins to relax (Maher, 1988).

MANAGEMENT SUGGESTIONS FOR TONIC BITE REFLEX

Suggest the following for the infant with tonic bite reflex:

1. After latching the infant on the breast, use the thumb or finger to press downward on the chin while the infant breastfeeds. Doing this throughout a breastfeeding session may allow the mother to nurse without discomfort (Maher, 1988).

2. A hungry infant may become tense and frantic while trying to latch on to the breast. For the infant with tonic bite reflex latch on while tense and frantic is even more difficult. The mother may need to express a small amount of breastmilk and give it to the infant before she offers the breast.

3. If the situation does not improve with management techniques and/or weight loss occurs, the mother may need to express her breastmilk and feed the infant using alternative methods until the clenching begins to relax.

Complementary and Supplementary Feeds

Complementary feedings are those given in addition to breastfeeding. Supplementary feedings are those feeds given that replace a breastfeeding. Routine complementary or supplementary feeds for the breastfeeding infant are unnecessary and not recommended unless there is a problem detrimental to the infant's well-being and it is medically indicated. The mother's breastmilk alone is a complete form of infant nutrition. Breastmilk meets all the infant's nutritional and fluid requirements. Research has shown that breastfed infants need no additional feeds, even in warmer climates (Goldberg & Adams, 1983). These additional or replacement feeds can interfere with the breastfeeding process and also affect the health of the breastfeeding mother and infant.

The routine use of complementary or supplementary feeds for the breastfeeding infant may easily destroy a successful breastfeeding relationship. Nipple confusion plays a part in this; but also the infant's hunger may be satisfied and cause him or her to go for longer stretches of time between nursing (AAP/ACOG, 1988). This in turn reduces the amount of stimulation on the nipple, which will contribute to a decreased milk supply. The relationship between the supplementary bottle offered to a breastfed infant and early weaning has been documented in studies (Ryan et al., 1990; Samuels, Margen, & Schoen, 1985).

Many justifications for supplementary and complementary feeds are not valid. If there is a medical indication for additional or replacement feeds, the mother should be instructed on breastmilk expression, to assist her in maintaining her milk supply, as well as alternative methods of feeding her infant other than artificial teats or bottles.

REASONS TO OFFER COMPLEMENTARY AND SUPPLEMENTARY FEEDS

The reasons given for offering supplementary and complementary feeds include the following:

1. *To detect a possible tracheoesophageal fistula* – Colostrum is a physiological secretion. It does not cause an irritating effect like a foreign substance. It is readily absorbed in the respiratory tree if aspirated (Lawrence, 1989).

2. *To treat or prevent hyperbilirubinemia* – Studies have shown that complementary and supplementary feeds do not prevent or "flush out" jaundice by reducing the bilirubin levels and may actually increase levels. Breastfeeding aids in the expulsion of meconium and decreases the incidence of hyperbilirubinemia (AAP & CPS, 1978; De Carvalho, Klaus, & Merkats, 1982).

3. *Not making enough milk* – A breastfeeding mother's milk production is greatly influenced by the introduction of additional or replacement feeds (Lawrence, 1989). Production is dependent on how often and how effectively the infant nurses. When receiving nutrition by means other than breastmilk, the infant may go for longer stretches between nursings and

take less milk from the breast when he or she does nurse, which leads to decreased breast stimulation and a decreased milk supply. The mother should be encouraged to breastfeed on demand, at least every two to three hours, for unrestricted time limitations. Wet diapers, although an effective tool for assessing intake once the mother is past the colostrum stage, should not be emphasized during the first few days because colostrum ingestion does not produce as many wet diapers. When complementary or supplementary feeds are medically necessary, the lactation consultant should work with the medical team to solve the problem. See Module 4, *The Management of Breastfeeding*, Chapter 2, for guidelines on the use of supplementary feeds in growth deficit.

4. *Hospital routine* – The mother whose infant is routinely getting complementary or supplementary feeds may perceive this as an unspoken message that her breastmilk alone is not enough to nourish her infant. This often leads to untimely weaning from the breast resulting from a decreased milk supply, as discussed above, or from nipple confusion (AAP & CPS, 1978; Bergevin, Dougherty, & Kramer, 1983).

5. *Medically indicated reasons* – If complementary or supplementary feeds are medically indicated, discuss various alternative feeding methods, other than the bottle, with the mother and physician. The breastfeeding mother should also be instructed on ways to maintain and increase her milk supply during this period.

POST-TEST

For questions 1 to 8, choose the best answer.

1. Changes in the taste of breastmilk

   A. may be caused by mastitis, malignancy, and menstrual cycle.
   B. may cause an infant to reject the breast.
   C. Both A and B.
   D. None of the above.

2. Position the infant at the breast so that

   A. his or her head is always in straight alignment with the body.
   B. the infant's ventral surface is against the mother's ventral surface.
   C. his cheek is turned toward the nipple.
   D. Both A and B.

3. Observe infants doing the following during a breastfeeding session:

   A. rooting, sucking, and burping.
   B. rooting, sucking, and swallowing.
   C. sucking, swallowing, and rejecting the breast.
   D. Both A and B.

4. Sucking difficulties in the premature infant may be due to

   A. developmental immaturity.
   B. neurological impairments.
   C. a delay in offering the breast.
   D. Both A and C.
   E. A, B, and C.

5. The dancer hand position is useful for the

   A. infant with a weak suck.
   B. infant with nipple confusion.
   C. infant with ankyloglossia.
   D. None of the above

6. Nipple confusion is best treated by

   A. giving all bottle feedings.
   B. feeding by alternative methods other than an artificial teat for the first day.
   C. ignoring the problem and continuing to offer the breast for feedings.
   D. offering the breast first and topping the feeding with a bottle.

7. When the infant sucks at the breast

   A. the tongue is extended over the lower alveolar ridge and flattened.
   B. the tongue is extended over the lower alveolar ridge and troughed.
   C. the tongue is rolled upward so that the frenulum is exposed.
   D. the tongue is retracted back in the mouth and flattened.

8. Which of these may lead to nipple confusion?
   A. Exclusive, frequent bottle feedings
   B. Alternating breast and bottle feedings
   C. Exclusive, frequent breastfeedings
   D. Both A and B.
   E. Both B and C.

For questions 9 to 14, choose the best answer from the following key:

A. Ankyloglossia   C. Tonic bite reflex
B. Tongue thrusting D. Weak suck

9. The breast continually falls out of the infant's mouth during a breastfeeding session.

10. The infants who most often present with this problem have a history of early introduction of artificial teats, are born prematurely, or are born with a neurological problem.

11. Use of the dancer hand position may prove very helpful.

12. A congenital syndrome.

13. Infant bites down on anything touching the inside of his or her mouth.

14. Frenotomy is one of the treatments used to correct this.

For questions 15 to 20, choose the best answer from the following key:

A. True   B. False

15. A hospital routine of offering free infant-formula gift packs to breastfeeding mothers may have a negative impact on a successful breastfeeding relationship.

16. Offering the breastfed infant complementary and supplementary feeds helps reduce jaundice by decreasing bilirubin levels.

17. Colostrum is a physiologic secretion and will not cause an irritating effect as will a foreign substance given to an infant to help detect a possible tracheo-esophageal fistula. It is readily absorbed in the respiratory tree if aspirated.

18. There is no reason for a breastfed infant to ever need complementary or supplementary feeds.

19. A breastfeeding mother's milk production may be greatly affected by the introduction of additional or replacement feeds.

20. Breastmilk does not completely meet the fluid needs of those infants living in warm climates.

References

Alper, JC (1983). Moist wound healing under a vapor-permeable membrane. *J Amer Acad Dermatol*, 8:3.

American Academy of Pediatrics (AAP), Committee on Drugs (1994). Transfer of drugs and other chemicals into human milk. *Pediatrics*, 93:137-50.

AAP, Committee on Nutrition, and Canadian Paediatric Society (CPS), Nutrition Committee (1978). Breastfeeding: A commentary in celebration of the international year of the child. *Pediatrics*, 62:591-601.

Amir, LH (1991). Candida and the lactating breast. *J Hum Lact*, 7:177-81.

Andrusiak, F, Larose-Kuzenko, M (1987). *The Effects of an Overactive Letdown Reflex*. Lactation Consultant Series, Unit No. 13. Wayne, NJ: Avery Publishing Group.

Ardran, GM, Kemp, FH, Lind, J (1958). A cineradiographic study of breastfeeding. *Br J Radiol*, 31:156-62.

Armstrong, HC (1990). *Lactation Management Topic Outlines*. Nairobi, Kenya: IBFAN Africa.

Auerbach, KG (1990). The effect of nipple shields on maternal milk volume. *JOGNN*, 19:419-27.

Bergevin, Y, Dougherty, C, Kramer, MS (1983). Do infant formula samples shorten the duration of breastfeeding? *Lancet*, 1:1148-51.

Clark, EW (1975). Estimate of the general incidence of specific lanolin allergy. *J Soc Cosmet Chem*, 26:323-25.

Clark, EW (1993). Lanolin Dermatological Safety and Benefits. *Medela Rental Roundup*, 10(3):6.

Clark, EW, Blondeel, A, Cronin, E, Oleffe, JA, Wilkinson, DS (1977). Lanolin of reduced sensitizing potential. *Contact Dermatitis*, 3:69-74.

Cobo, E (1973). Effect of different doses of ethanol on the milk ejection reflex in lactating women. *Am J Obstet Gynecol*, 115:817-21.

Conner, AE (1979). Elevated levels of sodium and chloride in milk from a mastitis breast. *Pediatrics*, 63:910-11.

Crase, B (1992). What's new about lanolin? *Leaven*, 28:5.

Cronenwett, L, Stukel, T, Kearney, M, Barrett, J, Covington, C, Del Monte, K, Reinhardt, R, Rippe, L (1992). Single daily bottle use in the early weeks postpartum and breastfeeding outcomes. *Pediatrics*, 90:750-66.

DeCarvalho, M, Klaus, MH, Merkatz, RB (1982). Frequency of breastfeeding and serum bilirubin concentration. *Am J Dis Child*, 136:737-38.

De Coopman, JM, Nehring, S (1993). *Breastfeeding Management for Health-Care Professionals*. Ann Arbor, MI: De Coopman.

Dilts, C (1985). Nursing management of mastitis due to breastfeeding. *JOGNN*, 14:286-88.

Dunkle, LM, Schmidt, RR, O'Conner, DM (1979). Neonatal herpes simplex infection possibly acquired via maternal breast milk. *Pediatrics*, 63:250-51.

Ellis, DJ, Livingstone, VA, Hewat, RJ (1993). Assisting the breastfeeding mother: A problem-solving process. *J Hum Lact*, 9:89-93.

Fleiss, PM (1980). Discussion on mastitis and acute and chronic illness. In: Lawrence, R (ed.), *Counseling the Nursing Mother on Breastfeeding*. Report of the 11th Ross Round Table on Critical Approaches to Common Pediatric Problems. Columbus, OH: Ross Laboratories.

Frantz, KB (1982). *Managing Nipple Problems*. Reprint No. 11. Franklin Park, IL: La Leche League International.

Goldberg, NM, Adams, E (1983). Supplementary water for breastfed babies in a hot and dry climate. *Arch Dis Child*, 58:73-74.

Goldsmith, HS (1974). Milk-rejection sign of breast cancer. *Am J Surg*, 127:280-81.

Hadley, SA, Fitzsimmons, L (1990) Nutrition and wound healing. *Top Clin Nutr*, 5(4):72-81.

Ham, AW, Cormack, DH (1979). *Histology*, 8th ed. Philadelphia: JB Lippincott.

Hazelbaker, AK (1993). *The Assessment Tool for Lingual Frenulum Function (ATLFF): Use in a Lactation Consultant Private Practice*. Master's thesis, Pacific Oaks College.

Heughan, C, Grislis, G, Hunt, TK (1974). The effect of anemia on wound healing. *Ann Surg*, 179:163-67.

Hewat, RJ, Ellis, DJ (1987). A comparison of the effectiveness of two methods of nipple care. *Birth*, 14:41-45.

Hole, JW (1981). *Human Anatomy and Physiology*, 2nd ed. Dubuque, IA: Wm. C. Brown Company.

Hoover, K (1992). *Nipple Thrush*. Paper presented at the International Lactation Consultant Association Conference, Chicago.

Horne, HW, Scott, JM (1969). Intrauterine contraceptive devices in women with proven fertility: A five-year follow-up study. *Fertil Steril*, 20:400-4.

Huggins, K, Billion, SF (1993). Twenty cases of persistent sore nipples: Collaboration between lactation consultant and dermatologist. *J Hum Lact*, 9:8.

Huml, SC (1993). Moist Wound Healing: Current Concepts in Treatment. Paper presented at the Association of Women's Health, Obstetrics, and Neonatal Nurses (AWOHNN) national conference.

Jenson, D, Wallace, S, Kelsay, P (1994). LATCH: A breastfeeding charting system and documentation tool. *JOGNN*, 23:27-32.

Johnston, HA, Marcinak, JF (1990). Candidiasis in the breastfeeding mother and her infant. *JOGNN*, 19:171-73.

Lauwers, J, Woessner, C (1989). *Counseling the Nursing Mother*. Garden City Park, NY: Avery Publishing.

Lawrence, RA (1989). *Breastfeeding: A Guide for the Medical Profession*, 3rd ed. St. Louis: Mosby.

Lawrence, RA (1994). *Breastfeeding: A Guide for the Medical Profession*, 4th ed. St. Louis: Mosby.

Leis, HP, Greene, FL, Cummarata, A, Hifler, SE (1988). Nipple discharge: Surgical significance. *So Med J*, 81:1, 20-26.

Levenson, SM, Seifter, E (1977). Dysnutrition, wound healing, and resistance to infection. *Clin Plast Surg*, 4:375-88.

LLLI News Release (November, 1993). *New Beginnings.*

Maher, SM (1988). *An Overview of Solutions to Breastfeeding and Sucking Problems*. Franklin Park, IL: La Leche League International.

Matthews, K (1988). Developing an instrument to assess infant breastfeeding behavior in the early neonatal period. *Midwifery*, 4(4):154-55.

McCormack, WM, Rosner, B, McComb, DE, Evrard, JR, Zinner, SH (1985). Infection with *Chlamydia trachomatis* in female college students. *Am J Epidemiol*, 121:107-15.

McDonald, RE, Avery, DR (1983). *Dentistry for the Child and Adolescent* (p. 95). St. Louis: Mosby.

McNeilly, AS, McNeilly, JR (1978). Spontaneous milk ejection during lactation and its possible relevance to success of breastfeeding. *Br Med J*, 2:466-68.

Medela (1993). Medela Product Information. McHenry, IL: Medela, Inc.

Mennella, JA, Beauchamp, GK (1991). The transfer of alcohol to human milk. Effects on flavor and the infant's behavior. *N Engl J Med*, 325:981-85.

Meyer, LJ, de Miranda, P, Sheth, N, Spruance, S (1988). Acyclovir in human breastmilk. *Am J Obstet Gynecol*, 158:586-88.

Minchin, MK (1985). *Breastfeeding Matters: What We Need to Know about Infant Feeding*. Victoria, Australia: Alma Publications and George Allen and Unwin.

Mohrbacher, N, Stock, J (1991). *The Breastfeeding Answer Book*. La Leche League International: Franklin Park, IL.

Monograph for Lanolin, Pharmacy Board Bulletin, U.S. Pharmacopeial Convention, April 10, 1992.

Moon, JL, Humenick, SS (1989). Breast engorgement: Contributing variables mendable to nursing intervention. *JOGNN*, 18:309-15.

Mulford, C (1992). The mother-baby assessment (MBA): An "Apgar score" for breastfeeding. *J Hum Lact*, 8:79-82.

Neifert, M (1992). Breastfeeding after breast surgical procedure or breast cancer. *NAACOGS Clinical Issues in Perinatal and Women's Health Nursing*, 3:673-82.

Neifert, MR, DeMarzo, S, Seacat, J, Young, D, Leff, M, Orleans, M (1990). The influence of breast surgery, breast appearance, and pregnancy-induced breast changes on lactating sufficiency as measured by infant weight gain. *Birth*, 17(1):31-38.

Neifert, MR, Seacat, JM (1986). A guide to successful breastfeeding. *Contemp Pediatr*, 3:1-14.

Neville, MC, Neifert, MR (1983). *Lactation: Physiology, Nutrition, and Breastfeeding*. New York: Plenum Press.

Newton, M, Newton, NR (1948). The let-down reflex in human lactation. *J Pediatr*, 33:698-704.

Niebyl, JR, Spence, MR, Parmley, TH (1978). Sporadic (nonepidemic) puerperal mastitis. *J Repro Med*, 20:97-100.

Notestine, GE (1990). The importance of the identification of ankyloglossia (short lingual frenulum) as a cause of breastfeeding problems. *J Hum Lact*, 6:113-15.

O'Callaghan, MA (1981). A typical discharge from the breast during pregnancy and/or lactation. *Aust NZ Obstet Gynecol*, 21:214-16.

Reilly, JJ, Gerhardt, AL (1985). *Modern Surgical Nutrition*. Chicago: Year Book.

Renfrew, M, Fisher, C, Arms, S (1990). *Bestfeeding: Getting Breastfeeding Right for You*. Berkeley, CA: Celestial Arts.

Riordan, J, Auerbach, KG (1993). *Breastfeeding and Human Lactation*. Boston: Jones and Bartlett.

Riordan, JM, Nichols, FH (1990). A descriptive study of lactation mastitis in long-term breastfeeding women. *J Hum Lact*, 6:53-58.

Ruberg, RL (1987). Role of nutrition in wound healing. *Surg Clin North Am*, 64:705-14.

Ryan, AS, Wysong, JL, Martinez, GA, Simon, SD (1990). Duration of breastfeeding patterns established in the hospital: Influencing factors. Results from a national survey. *Clin Pediatr*, 29(2):99-107.

Samuels, SE, Margen, S, Schoen, EJ (1985). Incidence and duration of breastfeeding in health maintenance organization population. *Am J Clin Nutr*, 42:504-10.

Schwartz, GF (1982). Benign neoplasms and inflammations of the breast. *Clin Obstet Gynecol*, 25(2):373-81.

Sharp, DA (1992). Moist wound healing for sore or cracked nipples. *Breastfeeding Abst*, 12:2.

Shrago, LC (1991). Engorgement reconsidered. *Breastfeeding Abst*, 11:1-2.

Shrago, LC, Bocar, DL (1990). The infant's contribution to breastfeeding. *JOGNN*, 19:209-15.

Spangler, A (1995). *Breastfeeding: A Parent's Guide* (p. 26). Atlanta, GA.

Spangler, A, Hildebrandt, E (1993). The effect of modified lanolin on nipple pain/damage during the first ten days of breastfeeding. *IJCE*, 8(3):15-19.

Tabar, L, Marton, Z, Kadas, I (1974). Galactography in the examination of secretory breast. *Amer J Surg*, 127:282-86.

Taddio, A, Klein, J, Koren, G (1994). Acyclovir excretion in human breast milk. *Ann Pharm*, 28:585-7.

Thomsen, AD, Espersen, T, Maigaard, S (1984). Course and treatment of milk stasis, noninfectious inflammation of the breast, and infectious mastitis in nursing women. *Am J Obstet Gynecol*, 149:492-95.

Utter, A (1992). Gentian violet and thrush. *J Hum Lact*, 8:6.

Vorherr, H (1992). *The Breast: Morphology, Physiology and Lactation* (pp. 220-26). New York: Academic Press.

Vorherr, H, Vorherr, UF, McConnell, TS, Goldberg, NM, Kornfeld, M, Jordan, SW (1974). Localization and origin of antidiuretic principle in para-endocrine-active malignant tumors. *Oncology*, 29:201-18.

Walker, M, Driscoll, JW (1989). Sore nipples: The new mother's nemesis. *MCN*, 14:260-65.

Weber, F, Woolridge, MW, Baum, JD (1986). An ultrasonographic study of the organization of sucking and swallowing by newborn infants. *Dev Med Child Neurol*, 28: 19-24.

Wei, SHY (1988). *Pediatric Dentistry: Total Patient Care.* Philadelphia: Lea & Febiger.

Wheater, PR, Burkitt, GH, Daniels (1979). *VG Functional Histology: A Text and Color Atlas.* New York: Churchill Livingstone.

Whitley, N (1974). Preparation for breastfeeding: A one-year follow-up of 34 nursing mothers. *JOGNN*, 7:44-48.

Woolridge, MW (1986). The 'anatomy' of infant sucking. *Midwifery*, 2:164-71.

Woolridge, MW, Fisher, C (1988). Colic, overfeeding, and symptoms of lactose malabsorption in the breastfed baby: A possible artifact of feeding management. *Lancet*, 2:382-84.

World Health Organization (WHO) (1990). Supporting breastfeeding: What governments and healthcare workers can do—European experience. *Int J Gyn Obstet*, 31 (Suppl)1:69-77.

ADDITIONAL READINGS

Alexander, JM, Grant, AM, Campbell, MJ (1993). Randomized control trial of breast shells and Hoffman's exercises for inverted and non-protractile nipples. *Br Med J*, 304:1030-32.

American Academy of Pediatrics (AAP), Committee on Fetus and Newborn/Committee on Infectious Disease (1980). Perinatal herpes simplex virus infections. *Pediatrics*, 66:147.

AAP and American College of Obstetricians and Gynecologists (ACOG) (1992). *Guidelines for Perinatal Care*, 3rd ed (pp. 121, 124). Elk Grove Village, IL: AAP.

American Dietetic Association (1987). Position paper on the promotion of breastfeeding. *J Am Diet Assoc*, 86: 1580-85.

Australian Lactation Consultant Association (ALCA) (1992). White spots (corpora amylacea). *ALCA News*, 3(3):8-9.

Basler, RS, Lynch, PJ (1985). Black galactorrhea as a consequence of minocycline and phenothiazine therapy. *Arch Dermatol*, 121:417.

Caldwell, K (1981). Improving nipple graspability for successful breastfeeding. *JOGNN*, 10:277-79.

Clay, LS, Billet, SS, Campbell, L, Glazer, R, MacInnes, M, Marchesi, W (1990). Chronic Moniliasis. *J Nurs Midwif*, 35(6): 377-84.

Copeland, CA, Raebel, MA, Wagner, SL (1989). Pesticide residue in lanolin. *JAMA*, 261:242.

Elliot, JP, Flaherty, JF (1983). The use of breast stimulation to ripen the cervix in term pregnancies. *Am J Obstet Gynecol*, 145:553-56.

Garrett, A, Ashworth, M (1996). Nipple shields: Insight from two experts. *Medela Rental Roundup*, 13(4), 6-7.

Huggins, K (1986). *The Nursing Mother's Companion.* Boston: Harvard Common Press.

Kesaree, N, Banapurmath, CR, Banapurmath, S, Shamanur, K (1993). Treatment of inverted nipples using a disposable syringe. *J Hum Lact*, 9:27-29.

Marmet, C, Shell, E, Marmet, R (1990). Neonatal frenotomy may be necessary to correct breastfeeding problems. *J Hum Lact*, 6:117-21.

Medela, Inc. (1993). New Pure-Lan 100—100% Pure Lanolin. *Medela Rental Roundup*, 103.

Newman, J (1990). Breastfeeding problems associated with the early introduction of bottles and pacifiers. *J Hum Lact*, 6:59-63.

Newton, NR, Newton, M (1950). Relation of the let-down reflex to ability to breastfeed. *Pediatrics*, 5:726-33.

Nikodem, V, Danziger, D, Gebka, N, Gulmezoglu, AM, Hofmeyr, GJ (1993). Do cabbage leaves prevent breast engorgement? *Birth*, 20:61-4.

Rosier, W (1988). Cool cabbage compresses. *Breastfeeding Rev*, May:28-31.

Skoog, T (1965). Surgical correction of inverted nipples. *J Am Med Wom Assoc*, 20:931-35.

Winchell, K (1992). Nursing strike: Misunderstood feelings. *J Hum Lact*, 8:217-19.

Woolridge, MW, Ingram, JC, Baum, JD (1990). Do changes in pattern of breast usage alter the baby's nutrient intake? *Lancet*, 336:395-97.

CHAPTER 3

Breastfeeding Techniques, Accessories, and Resources

SECTION A

Expression, Collection, and Storage of Breastmilk

Jan B. Simpson, RN, BSN, IBCLC

LEARNING OBJECTIVES

At the completion of this section, the learner will be able to do the following:

1. Discuss and demonstrate the removal of breastmilk using the Marmet technique for the manual expression of breastmilk.
2. Discuss the four basic categories of breast pumps available for the mechanical expression of breastmilk, stating when each may be appropriate.
3. Identify and discuss features and characteristics of the numerous breast pumps available on the market.
4. Provide instructions and recommendations for the mother using a breast pump.
5. Provide instructions and guidelines for the collection, storage, and preparation of expressed breastmilk.
6. Discuss the benefits of human milk banking.

OUTLINE

I. Expression of Breastmilk

   A. Manual expression
      1. The Marmet Technique
      2. Hand-expression funnel

   B. Mechanical expression
      1. Basic pump categories
      2. Pumping suggestions
      3. Bilateral pumping (double pumping)

PRE-TEST

For questions 1 to 11, choose the best answer.

1. The Marmet Technique for manual expression of breastmilk includes
   A. massaging and stroking the breasts.
   B. shaking the breasts.
   C. expressing the breastmilk using a wavelike motion with the fingers.
   D. All of the above.
   E. Both B and C.

2. When manually expressing breastmilk, the position of the fingers should be
   A. on the areola, at the base of the nipple.
   B. on the nipple.
   C. approximately 1 to 1½ inches back from the nipple.
   D. approximately 1 to 1½ inches back from the areola edge.

3. The use of a manually operated breast pump is most appropriate for all of the following situations except:
   A. occasional pumping needs.
   B. long-term mother–infant separation.
   C. for collection of breastmilk.
   D. short-term mother–infant separation.

4. A mother approaches you for advice regarding the type of breast pump she should use while her infant remains hospitalized in the intensive care nursery over the next two months. You recommend
   A. a battery-operated breast pump from the department store.
   B. a manually operated breast pump.
   C. a fully automatic electric breast pump.
   D. that she not breastfeed due to the long-term separation she is facing.

5. Prior to pumping her breasts during a break at work, Ms. Jones assists her milk-ejection reflex by all of the following except

   A. breast massage.
   B. calling the sitter to check on her infant.
   C. cool cloth compresses.
   D. looking at a photo of her infant.

6. Ms. Smith's infant was born at 31-weeks gestation. When discussing breast pumping with her, you encourage her to pump

   A. every two hours around the clock.
   B. every three to four hours around the clock.
   C. a minimum of five times to as many as eight times in 24 hours for 20 combined minutes each session.
   D. every 4 hours during waking hours only.

7. Bilateral pumping is defined as

   A. using two small battery-operated pumps simultaneously.
   B. pumping on one breast while feeding the infant on the other breast.
   C. using an adapter kit for an electric breast pump that allows you to pump both breasts simultaneously.
   D. Both A and C.

8. Using a glass container for storing expressed breastmilk

   A. is not recommended due to the adherence of leukocytes to the glass.
   B. is recommended as the best way to store breastmilk to be used within 24 hours.
   C. is OK if breastmilk is going to be frozen. The leukocytes are destroyed by the process of freezing.
   D. Both A and C.
   E. Both B and C.

9. When storing breastmilk at home, the container should always include

   A. the date and time pumped.
   B. the mother's name.
   C. any medications the mother is taking.
   D. foods the mother has eaten in the past 24 hours.

10. A _____ is an appropriate container for storing frozen breastmilk.

    A. freezer bag made from polyethylene or polyethylene with an outer coating of nylon or polyester
    B. plastic 80-ml storage bottle with artificial teat (bottle nipple) fitted securely on top with plastic covering
    C. single, presterilized bottle liner bag with twist-tie closure
    D. All of the above.

11. When storing breastmilk for the young infant,

    A. store in two- to three-ounce portions. This allows for quick defrosting and preparation and discourages waste.
    B. store in large bags that will hold at least six ounces.
    C. store in ½-ounce to 1-ounce servings. This is all the young infant requires at any one feeding.
    D. store one ounce per one kilogram of infant's body weight.

For questions 12 to 16, choose the best answer from the following key:

A. 12 hours   D. 2 weeks
B. 4 to 24 hours   E. 3 to 4 months
C. 8 days   F. 30 minutes

12. Breastmilk may stay refrigerated for _____.

13. Colostrum may remain at room temperature for _____.

14. Breastmilk may remain frozen in a freezer box located inside the refrigerator for _____.

15. Breastmilk may remain frozen in a refrigerator freezer for _____.

16. Mature milk may remain at room temperature for _____.

For questions 17 to 20, choose the best answer from the following key:

A. True   B. False

17. If stored breastmilk appears slightly blue or yellow in color, it should be discarded and not given to the infant.

18. If the breastmilk separates into milk and cream after being stored, the cream portion should be spooned off and removed before feeding it to the infant.

19. Expressed breastmilk collected at different times of the day may be combined if both are cooled.

20. Microwaving breastmilk is OK for defrosting and warming breastmilk prior to giving it to the infant.

Expression of Breastmilk

In many situations, it is important for a lactating mother to express breastmilk. Several methods of milk removal can be recommended, depending on the length of time the mother will need to express her breastmilk and the situation the mother will be in to pump. Manual expression is a very efficient method of removing breastmilk. A mother may also be very successful at expressing her milk with a breast pump if proper instructions and supervision are given.

MANUAL EXPRESSION OF BREASTMILK

Manual expression is a practical and effective technique for obtaining breastmilk. Some mothers find it just as productive as a pump, or even more productive, after they have mastered the technique and have become comfortable with it. Different hand positions and techniques can be used to express breastmilk. Encourage the mother to use what works best for her. The mother will need to experiment with applying pressure to the lactiferous sinuses to determine the finger placement most effective for milk removal.

THE MARMET TECHNIQUE

The Marmet Technique of hand expression was developed by Chele Marmet, a lactation consultant and director of The Lactation Institute in Encino, California. The Marmet Technique combines massage, stroking, and shaking the breasts with the technique of expressing the breastmilk by creating a wavelike motion with the fingers. This combination assists in stimulating the milk-ejection reflex and emptying the lactiferous sinuses. An excerpt from The Lactation Institute's pamphlet* follows.

The Marmet Technique of Manual Expression

EXPRESSING THE MILK:
DRAINING THE MILK RESERVOIRS
1. **POSITION** the thumb and first two fingers about **1" to 1½" behind the nipple**.
   - Use this measurement, which is not necessarily the outer edge of the areola, as a guide. The areola varies in size from one woman to another.
   - Place the thumb pad above the nipple and the finger pads below the nipple, forming the letter *C* with the hand, as shown in Figure 3A–1.
   - Note that the fingers are positioned so that the milk reservoirs lie beneath them.
   - Avoid cupping the breast, as shown in Figure 3A–2.

Figure 3A–1
Correct "C" fingers' position.

Marmet, C (1988). Manual Expression of Breastmilk—Marmet Technique. Copyright 1978, revised 1979, 1981, and 1988 by Chele Marmet. Used with permission of Chele Marmet and The Lactation Institute (16430 Ventura Blvd., Suite 303, Encino, CA 91436, USA: 818-995-1913).

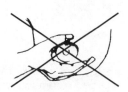

Figure 3A–2 Incorrect "C" fingers' position.

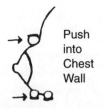

Push into Chest Wall

Figure 3A–3 Push on chest wall.

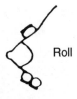

Roll

Figure 3A–4 Use a rolling motion.

2. **PUSH** straight into the chest wall, as shown in Figure 3A–3.
   - Avoid spreading the fingers apart.
   - For large breasts, first lift and then push into the chest wall.
3. **ROLL** thumb and fingers forward as if making thumb and fingerprints at the same time.
   - The **rolling motion** of the thumb and fingers compresses and empties the milk reservoirs without hurting sensitive breast tissue.
   - Note the moving position of the thumbnail and fingernails in the illustration (Figure 3A–4).
4. **REPEAT RHYTHMICALLY** to drain the reservoirs.
   - Position, push, roll; position, push, roll.
5. **ROTATE** the thumb and finger position to milk the other reservoirs. Use both hands on each breast. These pictures show hand positions on the right breast (see Figure 3A–5).

AVOID THESE MOTIONS
   - **Avoid squeezing** the breast. This can cause bruising.
   - **Avoid pulling** out the nipple and breast. This can cause tissue damage.
   - **Avoid sliding** on the breast. This can cause skin burns.

ASSISTING THE MILK EJECTION REFLEX: STIMULATING THE FLOW OF MILK
1. **MASSAGE** the milk-producing cells and ducts (see Figure 3A–6).
   - Start at the top of the breast. Press firmly into the chest wall. Move fingers in a circular motion on one spot on the skin.
   - After a few seconds, move the fingers to the next area on the breast.
   - **Spiral** around the breast toward the areola using this massage.
   - The motion is similar to that used in a breast examination.
2. **STROKE** the breast area from the top of the breast to the nipple with a light **tickle-like** stroke (see Figure 3A–7).
   Continue this stroking motion from the chest wall to the nipple around the whole breast.
   This will help with relaxation and will help stimulate the milk ejection reflex.
3. **SHAKE** the breast while leaning forward so that gravity will help the milk eject (see Figure 3A–8).

PROCEDURE
This procedure should be followed by mothers who are expressing in place of a full feeding and those who need to establish, increase, or maintain their milk supply when the baby cannot breastfeed.
   - Express each breast until the flow of milk slows down.
   - Assist the milk ejection reflex (massage, stroke, shake) on both breasts. This can be done simultaneously.

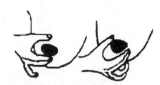

Right Hand

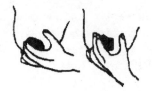

Left Hand

Figure 3A–5
Use rotating motion to express milk.

Massage

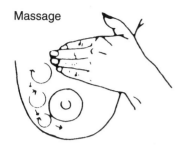

Figure 3A–6
Proper massage technique.

Stroke

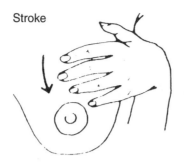

Figure 3A–7
Proper stroking motion.

Shake

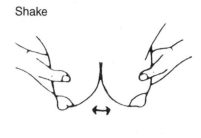

Figure 3A–8
Shaking helps.

- Repeat the whole process of expressing each breast and assisting the milk ejection reflex once or twice more. The flow of milk usually slows down sooner the second and third time, as the reservoirs are drained.

TIMING
The ENTIRE PROCEDURE should take approximately 20 to 30 minutes.
- Express each breast 5 to 7 minutes.
- Massage, stroke, shake.
- Express each breast 3 to 5 minutes.
- Massage, stroke, shake.
- Express each breast 2 to 3 minutes.

Note: If the milk supply is established, use the times given only as a guide. Watch the flow of milk and change breasts when the flow gets small. If little or no milk is present yet, follow these suggested times closely.

Hand-Expression Funnel

The manual expression of breastmilk is a natural process that can be done with any type of collection container. Manufacturers have developed a funnel to make the process of collection even easier, however, and to reduce worries about waste and mess. One such funnel is the Hand Expression Funnel by Medela, Inc. (see Figure 3A–9). The Hand Expression Funnel has a large opening to collect the sprays of milk as the woman expresses her milk by hand. The funnel is deep, with a rim that is rolled inward, which helps eliminate waste and keeps surrounding areas clean. As a less expensive alternative, a flexible bowl or cup can be used to collect breastmilk during the expression process.

Figure 3A–9
Hand-Expression Funnel.
Source: Copyright © 1994 Medela®, Inc., McHenry, IL. Reprinted with permission.

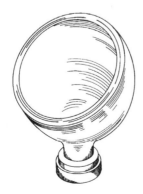

MECHANICAL EXPRESSION

Basic Pump Categories

There are many types and brands of breast pumps available for consumer purchase. The lactating mother should be carefully evaluated and supervised when breastfeeding accessories like these are being used to ensure proper usage. Problems should be corrected and breast pumps used only when necessary and required. The infant at the breast is more effective than even the best pump and the lactation consultant should not recommend a pump over the infant unless warranted by a medical or social situation.

Breast pumps can be divided into four basic categories. The following is a listing of the four categories with benefits of use listed below each:

1. Manually Operated Breast Pumps
   - Short-term separations
   - Occasional pumping needs
   - For collection and storage of breastmilk
2. Battery-Operated Breast Pumps
   - Short-term separations
   - Occasional pumping needs
   - For collection and storage of breastmilk
3. Electric Breast Pumps/Semiautomatic Diaphragm
   - Short-term separations
   - Occasional pumping needs
   - For collection and storage of breastmilk
   - Single or bilateral pumping capabilities
4. Electric Breast Pumps/Automatic Piston and Diaphragm
   - Long-term separations
   - Initiation of breastmilk supply if breastfeeding is delayed following birth
   - Maintenance of breastmilk supply if breastfeeding is temporarily interrupted
   - Collection and storage of breastmilk (ideal for mothers who work—convenient/fast)
   - Single or bilateral pumping capabilities

Pumping Suggestions

Although there are breast pumps of many different makes and models available, some basic pumping pointers and tips may be used with most of them to assist the mother in obtaining the greatest yield of milk during her pumping time:

1. Read pump instructions.
2. Make sure breast pump parts are properly cleaned and sterilized as indicated.
3. Wash hands prior to handling the breasts, breastmilk, or breast pump.
4. Massaging the breast, applying warm water or warm compresses to the breast, looking at a photo of the infant, and thinking about the infant are some things that the mother may do to facilitate the milk-ejection reflex. The smell of clothing the infant wears can elicit a milk-ejection reflex in some women.

5. The mother should make her pumping environment comfortable. Having something to drink or read, or listening to soothing music, may make the session more relaxing. Pillows for support are often helpful.

6. Moisten the collection cup (flange) of the breast pump to help obtain a better seal on the breast.

7. Position the nipple in the center of the collection cup (flange). Operate the breast pump according to the manufacturer's instructions.

8. If using a breast pump with a suction strength control regulator, always start on the lowest setting, slowly moving the suction strength up to the level of comfort.

9. Some breast pumps require the suction to be released by the mother using her finger to press a bar or button. If this type is being used, instruct the mother not to hold the created negative pressure for long periods of time because this can be extremely damaging to the nipple. She should attempt to mimic the infant's suck–release rhythm by holding the negative pressure (suction) approximately one to three seconds. She should read the pump manufacturer's instructions for recommendations regarding the use of a particular breast pump.

10. When unable to pump both breasts simultaneously, switch pumping—alternating the breast being pumped several times—will sometimes assist the mother in obtaining a higher milk yield.
    a. Pump approximately five to seven minutes on each breast or until the flow slows.
    b. Begin again on the first breast pumped. Pump three to five minutes on each breast.
    c. Again, go to the first breast pumped, and pump two to three minutes, ending with two to three minutes on the second breast.

11. Total pumping time is usually approximately 20 to 30 minutes unless the mother is double pumping, which may be completed in 10 to 15 minutes.

12. If possible, pump breastmilk into the storage container. If this is not an option, the expressed milk should be carefully poured into a sterile container and stored.

13. Pumping frequency varies according to the situation. If the mother has to be away from the infant, she should try to establish a routine that would be similar to that of his or her feeding—every two to three hours. If the infant is premature or ill, pumping the breasts at least five times in a 24-hour period, with a total pumping time that surpasses 100 minutes, is necessary to maintain optimal milk production (Hopkinson, Schanler, & Garza, 1988). Most lactation consultants recommend eight to twelve pumping sessions in order to establish a good milk supply. If the infant will remain hospitalized for several months and is being maintained on total parenteral nutrition (TPN), the mother can eliminate the pumping sessions in the middle of the night until enteral feedings are begun.

14. Follow the manufacturer's instructions for proper cleaning of the pump. Breast pump parts should be rinsed with warm water following each use and then washed according to instructions as soon as possible.

Bilateral Pumping (Double Pumping)

Another option for the mother to consider when deciding on a breast pump is bilateral pumping, pumping both breasts simultaneously. This can be done by using two small battery-operated pumps simultaneously or by purchasing a double-pumping adapter kit that is used with a large, fully automatic breast pump. Bilateral pumping has many benefits, including the following:

1. Decreases pumping time by half
2. Raises serum prolactin levels (Neifert & Seacat, 1985)
3. Increases the average amount of milk obtained in a pumping session
4. Helps maintain lactation for longer periods of time

Mothers who may especially benefit from bilateral pumping include mothers who have infants in high-risk nurseries, mothers who are separated from their infants for long periods of time, mothers trying to build up their milk supply, and working mothers. Any mother who is pumping would benefit and enjoy the luxury of a double-pumping system.

A new feature introduced by pump companies is the ability for the mother to vary the cycling rhythm to her own special needs. Cycling frequency can be set between 30 to 60 times a minute. This new feature substantially changes electric-pump capabilities. The Medela Lactina Select features adjustable pumping speed (see Figure 3A–10). Speed is adjusted by a small dial on the front of the pump. Settings range from one to seven, with one corresponding to 42 cycles per minute and seven to 60 cycles per minute. The Egnell Elite features an infinite range of safe cycle and suction levels with the unique capability of adjusting each function independently. It combines variable suction levels (0–250 mm HG) along with adjustable suction cycles (30–60 cycles per minute).

BREAST PUMP BRANDS

A variety of breast pumps are available to the consumer. Different manufacturers offer different styles of pumps, with different options, to meet the needs of the breastfeeding duo. Because of the wide variety of breast pumps on the market, individual discussion of each pump is not practical for this publication's purpose. *The Breastfeeding Product Guide* (Frantz, 1994) provides in-depth information on pumps. Table 3A–1 contains a brief description of a selected variety of breast pumps based on information currently available.

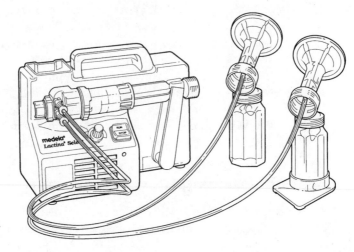

Figure 3A–10

An electric breast pump with bilateral pumping capabilities.

Source: Lactina® Breast Pump. Lactina is a registered trademark of Medela, Inc., McHenry, IL. Reprinted with permission.

Table 3A-1   Breast Pump Brands and Features

MANUALLY OPERATED BREAST PUMPS

Ameda/Egnell Cylinder Hand Breast Pump (Hollister, Inc.)	• Cylinder pump • Vertical pulling action/two-hand operation • Pump's breast shields are provided in two sizes: normal and large. • Milk pumped into cylinder that can be converted into bottle. • Dishwasher-safe • Milk contamination possible due to design of pump
Ameda/Egnell One-Hand Breast Pump (Hollister, Inc.)	• Small, light (4 ounces or 113 grams), portable • One-hand operation; allows mother to double-pump with two pumps or to operate while feeding on one breast • Can pump directly into a Mother's Touch freezer bag or bottle • Includes Flexishield nipple stimulator, designed to increase milk flow and volume • Dishwasher-safe • Suction adjusted by hand motion (varying speed and intensity) • Design minimizes possibility of milk contamination
Avent Manual Breast Pump (Cannon Babysafe, Ltd.)	• One-hand operation • Squeeze-trigger handle creates the suction • Vacuum-release valve is controlled by finger • Has a thin membrane that fits over the collection cup (flange) • Must use Avent bottle to operate pump
Comfort Plus Manual Breast Pump (Omron Healthcare, Inc.) **Ross Manual Breast Pump**	• Linear cylinder • Milk is collected in the cylinder. • Two-hand operation • Not autoclavable • Ross breast pump has two collection cups. Comfort Plus manual breast pump has collection cups with adapter inserts. • Potential problem of milk splashing from pump to breast as milk moves around with each stroke of the pump • Cylinders may come apart while pumping if long strokes are used; collected milk would then be wasted.
Precious Care Manual Breast Pump (Gerber Products Company)	• Collection cup is angled for downward pull. • Two-hand operation • Autoclavable
Evenflo Deluxe Manual Breast Pump	• Cylinder • Two-hand operation • Difficult upward arm pull on top cylinder, which can pull completely out • Not autoclavable • Milk is collected in baby bottle.
Little Hearts Manual Breast Pump (Medela, Inc.)	• Horizontal pulling action/two-hand operation • Milk is collected in separate bottle • Autoclavable, dishwasher-safe
Loyd-B Manual Breast Pump (Lopuco, Ltd.)	• Squeeze-trigger handle for creating suction and a finger-controlled release valve for releasing suction • Two-hand operation • Mothers with small hands may have difficulty using. • Milk is collected into collection jar the size of baby food jar. • Glass and plastic collection cups are available. • Two sizes of collection cups are available. • Requires mother to regulate suction and release and requires more strength to operate than other hand pumps.
Medela Manual Breast Pump	• Cylinder pump • Horizontal pulling action/two-hand operation • Milk is collected in separate baby bottle.

continued

Table 3A–1   Breast Pump Brands and Features   *continued*

Medela Manual Breast Pump *cont.*	• Universal threads allow use with various type bottles • The only physiological action manual pump available (automatic suck/release/relax) • Three adjustable, safe vacuum levels (220 mm Hg) • Autoclavable/dishwasher-safe • Design minimizes milk contamination • Interchangeable parts allow easy conversion for use with piston electric pump, Lactina electric pump, or mini-electric pump • Adapter for collection cup • Spring Express feature reduces arm fatigue.
Medela Pedal Pump	• Light (5 pounds or 2268 grams) and quiet • No electrical outlet needed • Large and bulky; not portable • Double-pumping collection kit attached to a specially designed wooden foot pedal • Powered by leg muscles • Mother regulates suction and release
Ora'lac Manual Breast Pump (Lunas Enterprises)	• These pumps are not recommended. • Mother sucks on plastic tubing to create the negative pressure for vacuum in the bottle • The strength of the mother's suck may limit the pressure buildup. • Collection cup is attached to tubing that also leads to the collection bottle • Can be used more discreetly than some pumps
Evenflo Bulb Manual Breast Pump	• Bulb and collection cup are located on top of collection bottle for squeeze action. • Poor suction capabilities • Unable to clean bulb properly • Opaque collection cup obstructs mother's view of nipple.
Davol Breast Pump **Rexall Breast Pump** **Barum Breast Pump** **Bittner Breast Pump** **Bittner Prima Breast Pump** **Goodyear Breast Pump**	• These pumps are not recommended. • Rubber bulb for squeeze action attached to plastic horn/collection cup • Has small reservoir for collection of breastmilk and must be emptied every few squeezes • Milk flows into bulb that is difficult to clean properly and may become contaminated, harboring bacteria. • Bulb is to be squeezed only partially and released. If squeezed all the way, bruising can occur. Great potential for breast tissue damage with use of these type pumps. • The Bittner Prima is glass with the bulb located over the reservoir. The Barum is also glass.

BATTERY-POWERED BREAST PUMPS

Egnell Lact-B Battery-Powered Breast Pump (Hollister, Inc.)	• Six-level suction adjuster allows mother to adjust for comfort. • One-hand operation • Lightweight (nine ounces) and portable • Includes adapter for use with an electric pump • Hard plastic flange with silicone Flexishield stimulator included as a liner • Requires two AA alkaline or rechargeable batteries • Collection cup has size adapter. • Suction must be released by user pressing bar on front of pump. • Can damage nipples if mother does not follow directions and pump is used improperly (i.e., holding negative pressure for extended time)
Gentle Expressions Battery-Powered Breast Pump (Graham-Field, Inc.)	• Lightweight (seven ounces) and portable • One-hand operation • Suction must be released by user pressing small button. • Vacuum adjusted by using a dial. • Requires two AA batteries or may be operated with AC adapter.

Table 3A–1   *continued*

	• Can damage nipples if mother does not follow directions and pump is used improperly (i.e., holding negative pressure for extended time) • Collection cup (flange) is made of hard plastic; two silicone liner inserts are available
Magmag Battery-Operated Breast Pump (Omron Healthcare)	• Lightweight (seven ounces) and portable • User releases suction by pressing a suction control/release valve • Collection cup with two size adapters • May be operated with AC adapter • Flushing system to keep motor free of clogs
Pigeon Pump & Feed (Pigeon Corporation)	• Lightweight (eight ounces) and portable • Suction must be released by user. • Steady buzz at 65 decibels • Battery- or AC adapter–operated
Evenflo Soft Touch Ultra	• Small, light • Quiet, operates at 54 decibels • Mother regulates suction-and-release, so takes practice to master • Limited cycling • Limited warranty
Little Hearts Breast Pumps (Medela, Inc.)	• Small, light • Autocycle pumping action • Batteries loaded through convenient zippered top • Separate AC transformer available • Adjustable suction levels
Medela Mini Electric Breast Pump (Medela, Inc.)	• Lightweight and portable • Has physiological autocycle action (an automatic suck–release–relax cycle) • Suck–release–relax cycles are created automatically at approximately every 1–1½ seconds (32 cycles per minute) • Adjustable vacuum strength levels • Universal threads for use with any type collection bottle • Special filter protects motor from overflows and serves as a bacteriological filter • Bottle stand included • AC or DC operation; can be used with two AA batteries or ordinary outlet electricity (adapter included with pump) • Collection cup (flange) is made of hard plastic • Adaptable to double pumping although alternates breasts pumped so not simultaneous double pumping
Precious Care Electric Breast Pump (Gerber Products Company)	• Lightweight and portable • Mother uses finger to create and release the continuous suction/vacuum. • Vacuum strength is not adjustable. • Collection cup is small and unusually shaped; it may be uncomfortable. • Hard and soft collection cups (flanges) available • Milk safety trap available

FULL-SIZE AUTOMATIC ELECTRIC PISTON BREAST PUMPS

Ameda/Egnell SMB/Lact-E (Hollister, Inc.)	• Suck and release action is automatic (48–60 times per minute). • Different settings control degree of suction • Two sizes of collection cup are available. • Collection cup (flange) is made of hard plastic; Flexishield silicone liner is available • Bilateral pumping converter is available. • Manufacturer services pumps • Heavy (SMB—22 pounds or 9980 grams; Lact-E—11 pounds or 4990 grams) • Quiet

continued

Table 3A–1   Breast Pump Brands and Features   *continued*

Medela Classic Electric Breast Pump 015	• Physiological autocycle action (automatic suck–release–relax action) • Preset pulsed suction • Different settings control degree of suction • One collection cup with adapter included • Collection cup (flange) made of hard, clear plastic • Bilateral pumping converter available • Manufacturer services pumps • Quiet • Heavy (16 pounds or 7258 grams)

MIDSIZE AUTOMATIC ELECTRIC PISTON PUMPS

Ameda/Egnell Lact-E Lite/Elite (Hollister, Inc.)	• Physiological autocycle action • Different settings control degree of suction • Lact-E Lite is preset at 48 cycles per minute. • Elite has adjustable cycling (30–60 cycles per minute). • On the Elite, settings to control cycle and suction are independently operated. • Electric-, battery-, and/or car cigarette lighter–powered • Bilateral pumping kit available (preassembled) • Closed system design minimizes milk contamination • Manufacturer services pumps • Lightweight (less than 7 pounds), portable, and quiet • To be used with Ameda/Egnell Hygienic Kit. • Light (6.5 pounds or 2949 grams)
Medela Lactina Electric Breast Pump 016	• Three models of Lactina are available: 016 Lactina Select with pumping speed control, Lactina Plus with internal transformer, Lactina Plus with external transformer. • PowerPak for operation with batteries or car cigarette lighter is available. • Physiological autocycle action (suck–release–relax action) is automatic. • Adjustable suction strength • Bilateral pumping converter is available. • Uses the Medela Manualelectric breast pump kit or the Universal Pumping System for collection and pump piston • Collection cup (flange) made of hard, clear plastic • Lightweight (Select is 5 pounds or 2268 grams), portable, and quiet • Travel case included

AUTOMATIC ELECTRIC DIAPHRAGM PUMPS

Medela Pump In Style Breast Pump	• Physiological autocycle action (suck–release–relax action) is automatic. • Adjustable vacuum • Uses standard electrical outlet with AC transformer; battery operation with optional PowerPak • Designer shoulder bag with adjustable straps conceals breast pump. • Two storage compartments—one with thermal foil lining to store milk and one to hold empty bottles, tubing, and accessories • Equipped for single- or double-pumping • Light (7 pounds or 3175 grams)
White River Electric Breast Pump 9050 (White River Corporation)	• Continuous vacuum • Fully automatic • Comes with carrying case • Flexible silicon collection cup • Double-pumping adapter kit available • Generates 30 cycles per minute maximum • Heavy (12 pounds or 5443 grams)

Table 3A-1 *continued*

SEMI-AUTOMATIC ELECTRIC DIAPHRAGM PUMP

Gomco (Model #1118) (Allied Healthcare Products)	• Continuous vacuum • Vacuum is created by a compressor. • Fingertip control for creating and releasing vacuum by placing finger over the suction inlet hole and removing it for suction release • Caution given to not overfill the collection cup or tip the cup toward the tubing connector on the breast shield cap to prevent aspirating milk into the tubing and filter • Glass flange and collection container • Allied Healthcare Products is the manufacturer and sells only to distributors
Gomco (Model #218) (Allied Healthcare Products)	• Continuous vacuum • Fingertip control for creating and releasing vacuum available • Includes an automatic mode that allows user to select duration of applied vacuum from 2 seconds to 30 seconds. Pump automatically releases vacuum for 4 seconds before vacuum suction is reapplied. • Vacuum time is set by turning timer knob. • Glass flange and collection container • Allied Healthcare Products is the manufacturer and sells only to distributors
Nurture III Electric Breast Pump (also marketed as the Double-Up Breast Pump) (Bailey Medical Engineering)	• Lightweight and portable • New collection cup is larger than earlier model, with a smaller nipple tunnel. • Mother uses finger to create and release the continuous vacuum/suction • Design protects motor from milk overflow and reduces possibility of milk contamination. • Single or bilateral pumping available
Schuco Electric Breast Pump #136 and #400 (Allied Healthcare Products)	• Lightweight and portable • Fingertip control for creating and releasing vacuum • Vacuum level is not adjustable. • Model #136 is larger and intended for hospital, physician's office, or home use. • Model #400 is smaller and more compact. It is designed for retail sale and for home use. • Model #136 has an exclusive bacteria filter to eliminate overflow and contamination by airborne bacteria. • Allied Healthcare Products is the manufacturer and sells only to distributors.

HOMEMADE MANUAL BREAST PUMP (JUICE JAR BREAST PUMP)

Select a wide-mouthed, quart-size glass jar to make a homemade manual breast pump. Choose a jar that has a smooth rim with no jagged or rough edges. Fill the cleaned jar with boiling water for approximately one minute. After pouring the hot water out of the jar, cool the rim of the jar with a cool, wet cloth. Moisten the breast with water and, with the mother leaning over the jar, place the breast into the mouth of the jar, forming a seal. Slowly cool the jar by wiping it with a cool, wet cloth. This will cool the air inside the jar, which will create a vacuum. The mother can use this method of emptying the breast without any direct contact with the nipple, which is helpful for women with severe nipple soreness (Neville & Neifert, 1983; Rees, 1977).

BREAST PUMP CARE AND CLEANING

The mother should always read the manufacturer's directions included with a manufactured breast pump on proper usage and cleaning. The general rule of thumb is that the pump parts that come into contact with the breast or breastmilk should be sterilized before the first use of the day and washed with hot, soapy water and rinsed thoroughly after each use. Mothers who are pumping milk at home for an infant in a neonatal intensive care unit may be asked to sterilize more often. Some manufacturers provide detailed instructions on how to autoclave pump kits. Pump parts are usually easy to clean. It is wise practice to wash and sterilize the parts of rental pumps with an antibacterial, antiviral disinfectant between users.

Collection and Storage of Breastmilk

There are many situations in which a mother may want or need to collect and store breastmilk. When a mother decides to express and store breastmilk, the following topics should be included in the care plan and discussed with the mother:

METHODS OF BREASTMILK EXPRESSION

A wide variety of expression methods are available to mothers today. A mother may choose the simplicity of manual expression or, depending on the situation, opt for a purchased or rented breast pump.

1. Manual expression
2. Manual breast pump
3. Battery-operated breast pump
4. Electric breast pump (fully automatic or semiautomatic and piston or diaphragm pump)
5. Double-pump system or single-pump system

The mother will need to explore the variety of expression methods available and find the one that is appropriate to her situation and that she is comfortable with, as well as what works best for her (see the beginning of this section on the manual expression of breastmilk).

LOCATION FOR EXPRESSION

The mother should be in as comfortable a location as possible when expressing her milk. Whether at home, work, school, or even in the car, being in as relaxed and comfortable an atmosphere as possible will assist the mother with her milk-ejection reflex. The mother can also try the following tips to help with collection:

1. Warm water on the breasts (basin, bath, shower, or warm compresses)
2. Breast massage
3. If away from the infant, look at a photo of the infant while expressing; think about the infant; call the caregiver and check on the infant

Many companies, large and small, now have a pumping room available for working mothers who are continuing to breastfeed after returning to work. These rooms offer privacy, comfort, electric breast pumps, a refrigerator for milk storage, and breastfeeding information.

STORAGE CONTAINERS

A variety of containers can be used to store expressed milk. For many years, it was believed best to avoid glass storage containers for fresh milk if at all possible because leukocytes adhere to glass. Leukocytes are especially important to infants who are ill; the benefit of their protective properties would be lost if expressed milk was stored in glass. However, Goldblum et al. (1981) showed that leukocytes detach from the glass over time and after 24 hours the fresh milk in glass had greater leukocyte concentration than the fresh milk stored in plastic. Paxson and Cress (1979) showed that leukocytes are destroyed by the process of freezing.

When milk is stored in glass and polypropylene bottles, there is a loss of sIgA to *E coli* by 20% to 30% at 24 hours. Plastic (polyethylene) bag storage results in an even greater loss of sIgA to *E coli* (60% decrease) in the first 24 hours (Goldblum et al., 1981). Therefore, when breastmilk is to be given within 24 hours (thus not frozen), use glass or polypropylene bottles. Glass is easy to clean (Pittard, Geddis, & Brown, 1991) and does not interact with fat-soluble nutrients (Garza, Hopkinson, & Schanler, 1986; Goldblum et al., 1981).

Williamson and Murti (1996) studied the effects of the type of container (glass vs. stainless steel), temperature, and time of storage on total cell count, cell viability, functions of milk cells, and immunoglobulins in human milk. This study confirmed that glass is the better storage container when compared to stainless steel. Glass yielded a higher percentage of free living cells in suspension after storage of milk. Milk stored in stainless steel containers showed a statistically significant reduction in total cell count ($p < 0.01$).

Storage time also appears to be a factor that influences phagocytic capability of milk cells. Short periods (7 hours) of storage have minimal detrimental effect on cellular functions and antibody content, but milk cell content and viability decline beyond 7 hours (Williamson & Murti, 1996).

The small plastic 80-ml collection bottles that are available in many hospital nursery facilities as well as through companies supplying breast pumps and breastfeeding accessories are excellent storage containers, provided they are made of polycarbonate (a clear, hard plastic) or polypropylene (a cloudy, hard plastic). The polypropylene bottles are autoclavable. It is imperative that they be secured with fitted lids and not with artificial teats, which do not provide a closed environment. A drawback to the use of plastic is the adherence of fat. Benefits include decreasing the possibility of breakage and thereby wasting the stored milk.

Milk-storage bags made especially to store expressed human milk are an alternative choice for long-term milk storage. They are presterilized, made of 100% polyethylene or polyethylene with an outer coating of nylon or polyester, and some are self-sealing. Bags that are 100% polyethylene should not be used for premature infants because secretory IgA antibodies have been shown to be reduced by 60% when stored in this material (Goldblum et al., 1981; Hopkinson, Garza, & Asquith, 1990). There is less of a loss of antibodies from milk stored in bags with a polypropylene inner layer or glass containers.

Bags sold as disposable bottle liners are also an easily accessible option, but they have drawbacks. Although they are presterilized, they are not as durable for freezing milk as bags made specifically for freezing. They do not come with closures, but can be easily closed with twist ties. Instruct the mother who chooses to use bottle liner bags to always double-bag her milk before freezing to allow for possible fractures in the bag caused by expansion of the milk as it freezes. Encourage her to place double-bagged milk upright in a large plastic container with a lid while storing in the freezer.

Some women using plastic storage bags have complained of milk with a bad odor and taste. Lipids also are known to change over long-term storage and may contribute to any rancidity of the milk. With long-term storage (greater than 6 months), polyvinyl-chloride from the bags may leach into the milk. Manufacturers of bags with either nylon or polyester outer layers claim an outer layer of these materials protects the milk from outside odors. There is no independent research to support this claim, however.

Placing the freezer bag in a cup or glass to provide support for the bag while filling it with human milk is helpful. Many of the pumps currently available allow the mother to pump directly into the storage bag. Instruct the mother to always label the containers of expressed milk with the date and time expressed. If the breastmilk will be transported elsewhere, such as to a hospital or to a caregiver, she will also need to include the infant's name. Some hospitals request that the mother include any medication she is taking or any illness she has when she labels the milk containers.

Storing expressed breastmilk in two- to three-ounce portions allows for quick defrosting and preparation for the infant, and also discourages wasting. Smaller amounts can be saved for the premature infant just initiating enteral feedings. If more milk is needed, it is easy to take more out of storage. Any breastmilk in the container that is not taken by the infant at that feeding must be discarded and not fed to the infant later. The accuracy of the printed markings on bags varies: the health-care provider should carefully measure the amount of milk given to an infant if specific amounts have been ordered for the infant. To feed the milk, the health-care provider will have to transfer the milk to a bottle, nursing supplementer, or other feeding device. These other devices can provide an accurate measurement. Breastmilk that has been defrosted should not be refrozen.

STORAGE-TIME GUIDELINES

There are a number of opinions regarding storage guidelines for expressed milk. Research-based guidelines indicate colostrum and mature milk are safe at room temperature for 12 and up to 24 hours, respectively. The actual temperature of the room determines the guidelines, with shorter guidelines recommended for higher room temperatures. See Table 3A–2 for specific storage-time guidelines.

PREPARATION OF EXPRESSED BREASTMILK

Mothers should be educated regarding the appearance and preparation of expressed milk that has been refrigerated or frozen. Many mothers are alarmed by the color of the milk. It is normal for the breastmilk to appear blue or yellow in color. Also, many dyes that the mother ingests may also change the color of the breastmilk. Milk that has been frozen often appears yellow. This does not mean spoilage unless it tastes or smells foul.

Another concern mothers may have is the noticeable separation of the breastmilk into milk and cream when it is stored. Reassure the mother that this is also normal and that she should gently shake the container of breastmilk to mix it before offering it to the infant.

Expressed milk collected at different times of the day may be combined if both are cooled. Never mix warm milk with frozen breastmilk.

Table 3A-2   Storage-Time Guidelines

ROOM TEMPERATURE

Colostrum—12 hours at 80.6 to 89.6°F (27 to 32°C)
Mature Milk—4 to 24 hours
   4 to 6 hours at 79°F (25°C)
   10 hours at 66 to 72°F (19–22°C)
   24 hours at 60°F (15°C)
Previously Frozen Breastmilk—1 hour at room temperature

REFRIGERATOR

Eight days at 32 to 39°F (0 to 4°C)
- If expressed milk is to be frozen, do so within the first 24 hours of refrigeration
- Place in coldest part of the refrigerator. Do not store in the door.
- Previously frozen breastmilk may remain in the refrigerator 24 hours

FREEZER BOX LOCATED INSIDE THE REFRIGERATOR

Two weeks

REFRIGERATOR/FREEZER

Three to four months

SEPARATE UNIT DEEP FREEZER (0°F)

Six months or longer

Sources: Barger & Bull, 1987; Hamosh, 1996; Nwankwo, 1988; Pardou, 1994; Pittard, 1985; Smith, 1992; Sosa & Barness, 1987.

Breastmilk that has been stored in the freezer can be defrosted in the refrigerator or under cool running tap water, then slightly warm running water. Breastmilk only needs to be room temperature before it is offered to the infant. Do not microwave or heat directly on the stove; either method may destroy components of the breastmilk and may burn the infant. Once defrosted, breastmilk keeps when refrigerated for up to 24 hours (Smith, 1992). Do not refreeze breastmilk, but it can be kept refrigerated once thawed.

TRANSPORTATION OF EXPRESSED BREASTMILK

If expressed breastmilk is transported to another location, such as a hospital or caregiver's, it should be done so on ice. The hospital staff or caregiver should transfer it directly to the freezer upon arrival if it is not going to be used within the next 24 to 48 hours. Check the policy for handling pumped breastmilk. Fresh breastmilk is preferred for preterm or sick infants and institutions vary on the length of time fresh breastmilk can be stored in the refrigerator. A small, portable cooler with ice or coolants is adequate for breastmilk transportation. Special cooler cases made especially for this purpose can also be purchased.

Human Milk Banks

A human milk bank is a place where human milk is compiled, stored, and distributed after being sold or donated by lactating mothers. Current guidelines deter the practice of paying donors. It is sometimes necessary to store breastmilk or use stored breastmilk due to health problems of the infant or problems that the mother is facing. All breastmilk stored in a milk bank is only dispensed by prescription for assistance in treating various medical problems or situations (Arnold, 1993a).

Milk donors are mostly mothers of lactating infants that oftentimes donate their surplus expressed breastmilk. On some occasions, the mother of an infant who has died will express her breastmilk and provide it as a donation, while she is working on decreasing her milk supply. Sometimes mothers who have given their infants up for adoption donate their expressed breastmilk (Arnold, 1993b).

Any mother who is willing to donate her expressed breastmilk must meet certain qualifications and health criteria established by the Human Milk Banking Association of North America, Inc. (HMBANA) and the USDA. She must be a healthy lactating woman and test negative for HIV-1 and HIV-2, syphilis, hepatitis-B surface antigen, and HTLV-1. She must not be harboring acute or chronic infections. She should not be taking drugs (including birth control pills, aspirin, and acetaminophen) or drink excessive alcohol (greater than 0.5 g/kg/body weight). She should not use tobacco (Arnold, 1991; Arnold, 1993a; Lawrence, 1989). All donors and all breastmilk are carefully screened to help assure that the donated breastmilk is safe for use (Arnold, 1993a). Milk donors may be temporarily eliminated from the program under certain conditions, such as having an acute infection (including monilial and fungal infections), following the administration of an attenuated virus vaccine, during an active infection of the herpes simplex virus or varicella zoster, while experiencing clinical mastitis, and for a twelve-hour period following the intake of alcohol. The milk donor may again begin her milk donation at the discretion of the milk bank director (Arnold, 1993a).

Reasons for infants to receive donor breast milk include prematurity, malabsorption, formula intolerance, immunologic deficiencies, postoperative nutrition support, HIV infection, lactation failure in the mother, death of the mother who has been breastfeeding, and adoption.

The U.S. Food and Drug Administration and the Centers for Disease Control highly recommend that breastmilk donated to human milk banks be heat-treated. Heat treatment destroys bacterial and viral contaminations in human milk. Valuable components that may be urgently needed by some infants are also destroyed during this process, however (Arnold, 1993a). In cases where the infant requires a fresh preparation of breastmilk that has not been heat-treated, parents or guardians must sign additional consent forms releasing the human milk bank from liability.

Several terms used to describe human milk preparations follow (Arnold, 1993a):

- Fresh-raw milk is milk that is stored continuously at approximately 4°C for no longer than 72 hours after expression.
- Fresh-frozen milk is fresh-raw milk that has been frozen and held at approximately –20°C for less than 12 months.

- Heat-treated milk is fresh-raw or fresh-frozen milk that has been heated to not less than 56°C and held for 30 minutes—Holder Pasteurization.
- Pooled milk is milk from more than one donor.

Table 3A–3 lists members of the HMBANA.

Table 3A-3   Milk Banks in the United States and Canada

Central Massachusetts Milk Bank at Memorial/Mass. Medical Center 119 Belmont St. Worcester, MA 01605	Darlene Breed, RN, BSN, IBCLC Coordinator Phone: 508-793-6005 Fax: 508-793-6593
Mothers' Milk Bank Columbia/Presbyterian/ St. Luke's Medical Center 1719 E. 19th Avenue Denver, CO 80218	Laraine Lockhart Borman, BA, IBCLC Director Phone: 303-869-1888 Fax: 303-869-2490
Lactation Support Service British Columbia Children's Hospital 4480 Oak St. Vancouver, BC V6H 3V4 Canada	Agi Radcliffe, RN, IBCLC Coordinator Phone: 604-875-2345, ext. 7607 Fax: 604-875-2349
Medical Center of Delaware Mothers' Milk Bank Christiana Hospital, 2-A, Room 2340 4755 Ogletown-Stanton Rd. P.O. Box 6001 Newark, DE 19718	Maggie Conant Coordinator Phone: 302-733-2340
Mothers' Milk Bank Valley Medical Center 751 South Bascom Ave. San Jose, CA 95128	Pauline Sakamoto, RN, MS Coordinator Phone: 408-998-4550 Fax: 408-885-7381-MMB
National Capital Lactation Center and Community Human Milk Bank Georgetown University Medical Center 3800 Reservoir Rd. NW Washington, DC 20007	Phone: 202-784-6455 Fax: 202-784-2505
National Office of the HMBANA 8 Jan Sebastian Way, #13 Sandwich, MA 02563	Lois Arnold, MPH, IBCLC Executive Director Phone: 888-232-8809 / 508-888-4041 Fax: 508-888-8050 milkbank@capecod.net
Triangle Lactation Center/ Mothers' Milk Bank Wake Medical Center 3000 New Bern Ave. Raleigh, NC 27610	Mary Rose Tully, MPH, IBCLC Coordinator Phone: 919-250-8599 Fax: 919-250-7749 dtully@ral.mindspring.com

Electromagnetic Fields
and Electric Breast Pumps

Standards have not been established for electomagnetic field (EMF) emissions from electric breast pumps. At the present time, it is not known if EMFs from the use of an electric breast pump pose a health risk, although questions have been raised and debated. This highly publicized debate centers around what level of exposure should be considered reasonably safe.

An independent study reported by Ameda/Egnell (now owned by Hollister, Inc.), the engineering firm of Packer Engineering (Naperville, IL), confirmed that Ameda/Egnell's electrically powered breast pumps exposed the user to a lower EMF than a leading competitor's pump. (For more information on this study, contact Hollister, Inc., at 800-323-8750.)

POST-TEST

For questions 1 to 10, choose the best answer.

1. Colostrum may be safely kept at room temperature for

    A. 30 minutes.
    B. 1 to 2 hours.
    C. 12 hours.
    D. 6 to 10 hours.

2. Mature milk may be kept safely at room temperature for

    A. 12 to 24 hours.
    B. 1 to 2 hours.
    C. 4 to 24 hours.
    D. 30 minutes.

3. Mature milk may safely remain in frozen storage in a refrigerator-freezer for

    A. one month.
    B. three to four months.
    C. six months or longer.
    D. two weeks.

4. Breastmilk may safely remain in storage in the refrigerator for

    A. two weeks.
    B. two days.
    C. eight days.
    D. five days.

5. Breastmilk may safely remain in storage in a freezer box located inside the refrigerator for

    A. two weeks.
    B. two days.
    C. two months.
    D. five days.

6. Breastmilk may safely remain in frozen storage in a separate-unit deep freezer at temperatures below 0°F

    A. for three to four months.
    B. for six months or longer.
    C. indefinitely.
    D. for one month.

7. To safely defrost breastmilk that has been frozen,

    A. microwave for no more than 45 seconds then shake the container.
    B. place the container in boiling water on the stovetop.
    C. hold under cool, running tap water.
    D. leave the container out on a counter overnight.

8. Once defrosted, breastmilk may be refrozen only if

    A. it has not been in frozen storage longer than 2 months.
    B. it has been defrosted for no longer than 2 to 4 hours.
    C. it has been defrosted for no longer than 1 hour.
    D. Breastmilk should never be refrozen.

9. Once defrosted, breastmilk may be refrigerated for up to
    A. 24 hours.
    B. 9 hours.
    C. 6 hours.
    D. 12 hours.

10. Ms. Smith tells you that she wants to express and store her breastmilk for when she returns to work. Your instructions to her include which of the following statements?
    A. Never combine breastmilk that you have pumped at different times of the day.
    B. It is OK to combine fresh, pumped breastmilk with frozen breastmilk.
    C. Expressed milk collected at different times of the day may be combined if both are cooled.
    D. If the breastmilk appears to have separated into cream and milk after being stored, discard it and do not offer it to the infant.

For questions 11 to 15, choose the best answer from the following key:

A. True   B. False

11. When manually expressing breastmilk, the fingers should be positioned on the areola at the base of the nipple.

12. Pumping the breasts bilaterally can raise serum protein levels.

13. A manually operated breast pump is the first choice of pumps for the mother of a premature infant who will be hospitalized for 1 to 2 months.

14. One pump is just as good as another for expressing breastmilk.

15. A plastic bag is recommended as the first choice for storing breastmilk for less than 24 hours.

For questions 16 to 20, match the method of breastmilk expression you would recommend most highly with each statement. Each answer may be used more than once or not at all.

    A. Manually operated breast pump
    B. Fully automatic electric piston breast pump
    C. Manual expression
    D. Battery-operated breast pump
    E. A, C, and D

16. Mother who wants to express her breastmilk and has severely cracked nipples.

17. Mother who wants to relactate.

18. Mother who is unable to breastfeed following birth because of the infant's medical complications. The infant is in the intensive care nursery and is unable to breastfeed at the present time.

19. Mother who is planning a dinner date and will be separated from her infant for two hours.

20. Mother who is planning to adopt an infant within the next one to two months and wants to breastfeed.

SECTION B

Breastfeeding Accessories, Devices, and Supplemental Techniques

Jan B. Simpson, RN, BSN, IBCLC

LEARNING OBJECTIVES

At the completion of this section, the learner will be able to do the following:

1. Identify situations in which the use of breast shells may benefit the breastfeeding mother and infant.
2. Discuss the dangers that accompany the use of nipple shields and provide instructions for correct usage if a nipple shield is used.
3. Identify a dimpled nipple and discuss the use of a dimple ring.
4. Provide recommendations to the mother who will be purchasing nursing bras and bra pads.
5. Provide data regarding creams and ointments for the breasts, discussing which type of creams and ointments to avoid and providing supportive rationales.
6. Discuss the role of the nursing supplemental device and identify situations in which the device could be beneficial.
7. Provide recommendations on the technique of finger feeding for nutritional supplementation.
8. Describe cup feeding as a technique for nutritional supplementation.
9. Describe the use of a periodontal syringe for providing nutritional supplementation.
10. Discuss the function of nursing stools and nursing pillows for the breastfeeding mother.
11. Discuss fashion options for the breastfeeding mother, offering recommendations.

OUTLINE

I. Accessories

    A. Breast shells

    B. Nipple shields

    C. Dimple rings

    D. Breast Leakage Inhibitor System

    E. Bra pads

    F. Nursing bras

    G. Engorgement bras

    H. Ice flowers

    I. Cabbage compresses

    J. Breast creams and ointments

    K. Nursing stools

    L. Nursing fashions

    M. Nursing pillows

    N. Baby carriers

    O. Scales

II. Nursing Supplementer Devices

    A. Axi-Care Nursing Aid

    B. Lact-Aid

    C. Supplemental Nursing System

    D. Starter SNS

    E. Supply Line

    F. D-I-Y nursing supplementer

III. Other Supplementing Techniques

    A. Finger feeding

    B. Periodontal syringe

    C. Cup feeding

PRE-TEST

For questions 1 to 10, choose the best answer.

1. Ms. Smith is 20-weeks pregnant with her first child. She plans to breastfeed, but discusses her concerns with you about her inverted nipples. She questions you about the possibility of wearing breast shells. Your recommendations include:

    A. Begin wearing breast shells as soon as possible.

    B. Begin wearing the breast shells during her last trimester.

    C. Wear the breast shells between feedings during the postpartum period.

    D. Both A and C.

    E. Both B and C.

2. Breast shells

    A. can cause plugged ducts and mastitis.

    B. are a quick fix-it for mothers with flat or inverted nipples.

    C. are the best way to treat sore nipples.

    D. All of the above.

3. Nipple shields

    A. decrease the amount of breastmilk the infant receives when nursing by 10–20%.

    B. can cause a decrease in the mother's milk supply due to decreased stimulation of the nipple and decreased compression of the areola.

    C. protect the nipple from any tissue damage.

    D. All of the above.

4. When choosing a bra pad, the mother should

    A. choose a pad that has a protective liner of plastic that will prevent leakage onto her clothing.

    B. choose a pad that is made of 100% cotton or all paper.

    C. avoid pads that are colored using dyes.

    D. Both A and C.

    E. Both B and C.

5. Which of the following nursing bras should be avoided?

    A. Nursing bra with plastic liners in the cups

    B. Nursing bra with underwire support

    C. Nursing bra with mid-cup seams

    D. All of the above.

6. You counsel a mother who is engorged. Among possible management suggestions, you suggest the use of

    A. cold compresses.

    B. ice flowers.

    C. engorgement bras.

    D. All of the above.

7. Topicals for the breasts should definitely be avoided if they contain

    A. anesthetics.

    B. alcohol.

    C. free-lanolin alcohol content greater than 6%.

    D. Both A and B.

    E. All of the above.

8. _____ is an appropriate topical for the breasts of a nursing mother.

    A. Aloe vera

    B. Vitamin E

    C. Masse' cream

    D. Mother's own breastmilk

    E. All of the above.

9. A _____ is a device that helps provide the infant with a supplement while the infant is sucking at the breast.

   A. bottle
   B. nursing supplementer
   C. lactation tubing
   D. Haberman feeder

10. Infants who may benefit from the use of a nursing supplementer include

   A. premature infants.
   B. infants with cleft lip or cleft palate.
   C. failure-to-thrive infants.
   D. Both A and C.
   E. A, B, and C.

For questions 11 to 15, choose the best answer from the following key:
   A. **If responses 1, 2, and 3 are correct.**
   B. **If responses 1 and 3 are correct.**
   C. **If responses 2 and 4 are correct.**
   D. **If all the responses are correct.**

11. Finger feeding

   1. is a method used to supplement nourishment to an infant while teaching the infant to nurse more effectively.
   2. may cause ineffective sucking.
   3. may be accomplished with a syringe, gavage tube, or plastic dropper.
   4. should always be done prior to offering the infant the mother's breast to ensure proper sucking.

12. When using tubing for finger feeding, the tubing should be

   1. taped to the nail of the smallest digit.
   2. taped far enough back on the digit so the infant does not pull the tape into his mouth.
   3. as large as possible.
   4. taped to the pad side of the digit closest in size to the mother's nipple.

13. If a plastic dropper is being used for finger-feeding, the caregiver should not force the supplement into the infant's mouth because that could cause

   1. bradycardia.
   2. gagging.
   3. reduced oxygenation.
   4. aspiration.

14. The periodontal feeding syringe

   1. is a tool used for supplementing nourishment to the infant while he or she is at the breast.
   2. is a tool used for supplementing nourishment to the infant while he or she is being finger-fed.
   3. has a curved tip.
   4. is a 20-cc syringe with a plunger for forcing the nourishment into the infant's mouth.

15. Cup feeding

   1. is a way to supplement nourishment for infants who are older than six weeks instead of using bottles.

2. is a method of feeding whereby the caregiver slowly tips the cup so that the milk is just touching the infant's lips, allowing the infant to use his or her tongue to obtain milk.

3. is a method of feeding whereby the caregiver removes the cup from the infant's mouth each time he or she stops sipping the milk.

4. encourages the infant's tongue to extend over the rim of the cup.

For questions 16 to 20, choose the best answer from the following key:

A. True   B. False

16. Using cups in supplementing does not make infants unable or unwilling to suck at the breast.

17. Any breastmilk that collects in the breast shell from leaking may be fed to the infant or stored for future use.

18. Nipple shields are contraindicated for treatment of sore nipples.

19. One periodontal syringe may be repeatedly filled as needed for use during one feeding session.

20. Dark-colored clothing tends to make spots that occur due to leaking less noticeable.

Accessories

With breastfeeding on the rise, so is the marketing of breastfeeding devices and accessories. Although some are useful and strongly promote continuation of the breastfeeding relationship, others are unnecessary and could result in overdependence on the device by the mother and possible premature weaning. The professional must consider the short- and long-term needs of the breastfeeding mother and infant when making recommendations that involve the use of any breastfeeding accessory. Such accessories should be used only when required and only in conjunction with professional advice and instruction on appropriate use.

BREAST SHELLS

Breast shells (also widely known as milk cups) are plastic, raised, and rounded shells that the mother may wear in her bra for multiple purposes (see Figure 2C–5 in Chapter 2 in this module for an illustration of breast shells). Depending on the situation, the mother may begin wearing the breast shells during the last trimester of her pregnancy or during the postpartum period between feedings.

The breast shells can be worn discreetly despite their appearance. The mother may need to wear a bra one cup size larger to help accommodate the breast shell comfortably. If breast shells are worn too snugly, the constant pressure on the breasts may cause plugged ducts or mastitis.

Each breast shell consists of an outer dome and an inner ring. The outer dome is made of a hard, plastic material. It may have several holes, a few holes, one small hole, or no holes at all. A dome with multiple air holes works best, because it allows more air to circulate under it. Outer domes with one or no holes may not allow ample drying of the nipples, which may lead to nipple soreness (Auerbach, 1987).

Two types of inner rings are available: one with small openings and one with large. Inner rings are available in the same hard, plastic material that outer domes are made of or in a soft, flexible silicon.

The mother who has flat or inverted nipples and chooses to wear breast shells for treatment (to help draw the nipples out) should ideally begin wearing them during the last trimester of pregnancy. She should wear inner rings with small openings. She should begin wearing them for short periods—approximately 6 to 10 hours a day, or to her level of comfort. She should not sleep in the shells. After the infant is born, the mother may wear the shells approximately 30 minutes prior to putting the infant to breast to help pull the nipple out, if necessary, or she may wear them between feedings.

A randomized, controlled trial of breast shells and Hoffman's exercises for inverted and nonprotractile nipples showed no benefit from either (Alexander, Grant, & Campbell, 1993). Many lactation consultants no longer recommend breast shells for inverted nipples.

Breast shells may be worn to help protect sore nipples and may aid the healing process. For this purpose, inner rings with large openings should be worn. Breast shells help protect sore nipples from the friction of the bra and prevent the bra from sticking if the mother's breast leaks and then dries. The large, multiple air holes allow air to circulate, helping keep the nipple area free from surface wetness and promoting the healing process. Shells should not be worn as a quick-fix for sore nipples, however. The best way to treat sore nipples is to look at the etiology and correct the problem—by assuring proper latch-on and proper positioning or correcting the improper suck of the infant.

Mothers who are engorged wear breast shells with the inner rings with small openings to help promote softening of the areola by leakage of breastmilk. If breast shells are worn for this purpose, however, caution should be used because more severe problems, such as plugged ducts and mastitis, may develop.

The manufacturer's instructions on the care of the breast shell should be followed. The general rule of thumb for care of breast shells is daily washing in hot, soapy water and sterilizing once a week. If a candidiasis of the nipple area is present, more frequent washing and sterilizing may be indicated. Any breastmilk that collects in the breast shells should be discarded: It is an excellent medium for bacterial growth and should never be given to an infant (Auerbach, 1987).

NIPPLE SHIELDS

Nipple shields, not to be confused with breast shells, are made to be worn over the mother's nipple during a feeding (see Figure 2C–6 in Chapter 2 in this module for an illustration of nipple shields). Today, nipple shields are made of milky rubber or silicone, but in the past they have been made of glass and even wood. Nipple shields are distributed to treat sore nipples and ungraspable nipples. They should be used as a comfort measure for sore nipples but not as a substitute for correcting the etiology of the sore nipples.

Routine use of nipple shields is not recommended. Common concerns include the potential for reduced milk flow and/or milk production, a decrease in the amount of milk available to the infant, an inadequate emptying of the breast with resulting plugged ducts or a reduced milk supply, and the possibility that the infant may imprint on the artificial nipple and that the mother may develop a dependence on the shield (Amatayakul et al., 1987; Auerbach, 1990; Garrett & Ashworth, 1996; Jackson, Woolridge, & Imong, 1987). See Table 2A–1 in Chapter 2 in this module for other concerns about nipple shield use.

The following are some problems associated with nipple shield use:

1. May cause improper positioning of infant at breast
2. May cause an ineffective sucking pattern
3. Decreases stimulation of the nipple/areola area, thus potentially affecting the release of prolactin and oxytocin
4. May contribute to slow weight gain in the infant
5. May damage nipple and areola tissue if used improperly
6. Infant's acclimation to the feeling of rubber or silicone in his or her mouth may cause refusal of the breast without the nipple shield
7. Predisposes the nipple to possible damage when the infant is put to breast without the shield in place, because he or she may learn to chew rather than suck

8. Sends an unspoken message to the mother that she is unable to breast-feed, or that her breast is inappropriate for breastfeeding, without the barrier of a nipple shield in place

Continuous use of nipple shields has been shown to decrease the amount of milk the infant receives from the mother. The thick gum rubber nipple shield decreases the milk intake by as much as 58% (Woolridge, Baum, & Drewett, 1980). The thin silicone nipple shield decreases the milk intake by as much as 22%, which is better, but still not good (Lawrence, 1992; Woolridge, Baum, & Drewett, 1980). Due to the decreased stimulation of the nipple and decreased compression of the areola the mother receives when using the nipple shield and the reduced amount of milk being taken from the breast, her milk supply may be drastically decreased. Because the silicone nipple shield is thinner and more flexible, the areola receives more stimulation and the mother's milk volume is not as depleted as with other types of nipple shields (Auerbach, 1990).

When use of nipple shields is deemed appropriate, great caution should be exercised. Instructions and demonstration on the proper use of nipple shields must accompany any distribution of the shield. Detailed charting on the reason the nipple shield was used and the instructions given to the mother is warranted.

When using a nipple shield, moisten the inside rim of the shield with breastmilk or water to help obtain a good seal. Minchin (1989) suggests applying a thin smear of lubricant or petroleum jelly to the underside rim of the nipple shield. The mother then rolls her nipple between her fingers to help it protrude as much as possible. She inverts the brim of the shield, as if to turn it inside out. Garrett and Ashworth (1996) recommend stopping when the diameter of the inside of the shield brim matches the diameter of the nipple. The crown of the nipple shield is then placed over the nipple. The brim of the shield is smoothed over the areola and held in place. The edge of the crown will press into the areola. By holding the brim against the areola and teasing the crown out from the breast, a suction forms, which pulls the nipple forward into the shield. The mother may find it helpful to tape the shield securely in place before beginning the feeding (Garrett & Ashworth, 1996).

Present the breast to the infant, using the C-hold support behind the nipple shield. Pull back on the shield to stretch it against the breast. The infant's tongue should be under the shield as much as possible. It may be necessary to apply pressure to the top of the shield's brim in order to help the infant latch on. Once the infant latches on and shows an exuberant suck and the mother's nipple is more formed, the nipple shield should be removed and the infant again latched-on so he or she can suck at the breast.

Use of the newer silicon shields has resulted in case reports of women successfully lactating using a nipple shield for an extended period of time. Infant output and weight gain can indicate whether the infant is receiving adequate breastmilk to support growth. The mother may or may not need to pump or manually express her breasts for extra stimulation. Eliminating the shield is an individualized process for each mother. When a mother is confident her infant is growing and exhibits a wide root with an extended tongue and her nipples are more protracted or the soreness has healed, the shield can be eliminated.

If the infant has become acclimated to the nipple shield, refuses to breastfeed without it, and is not gaining weight well, requiring supplementation, weaning from the shield may be indicated. If the mother is using a gum rubber nipple shield, change to a silicone shield, which is thinner and more flexible. Some lactation consultants cut the tip of the shield as a weaning measure, but many now feel this is unnecessary. But when an infant refuses other weaning techniques, it may be necessary to cut the tip of the shield. Cut off the tip of the nipple shield to help enable a higher milk flow to the nursing infant, while beginning to expose more breast. (Suggestion: Turning a silicone shield inside out before cutting the tip off helps prevent a rough, raw edge from being presented to the infant.) Use the nipple shield very briefly (a few seconds), then remove it, and place the infant directly on the breast. A feeding-tube device that is taped directly to the areola and delivers a supplement may entice the infant and assist in adapting him or her to the breast more quickly (Walker & Auerbach,1993).

DIMPLE RINGS

When a nipple is dimpled, the tip folds inward, making a fissure. Sore and bleeding nipples may result. Breast shells may not correct a dimpled nipple. The dimple ring assists in holding the dimpled portion of the nipple outward in an exposed position so it can dry and healing can take place (Marmet & Shell, 1987). The dimple ring is made of a circular fabric with a hole for the nipple.

BREAST LEAKAGE INHIBITOR SYSTEM

The *blis*, Breast Leakage Inhibitor System, produced by Prolac, Inc., is a newly developed breastfeeding management tool to control leakage. It is designed to rest against the mother's nipple, creating enough pressure to inhibit leakage following a milk-ejection reflex. The *blis* shield is worn inside the bra, with the concave nipple of the shield placed in line with the woman's nipple. The *blis* pad is worn between the breast and shield. The *blis* can be used in various situations in which leakage is a problem, such as:

- when mother is away from her infant
- between feedings
- when nursing or expressing one breast, the shield may be worn on the other
- when exercising
- during intercourse

The *blis* should not be worn if:

- nipples are cracked or sore
- woman has, or is prone to having, plugged ducts or mastitis
- nipples are inverted

BRA PADS

Mothers may choose to use bra pads for protection against breastmilk leakage onto their clothing. There are many types of bra pads on the market. Disposable pads, reusable pads, and homemade pads all serve the purpose; however, there are some features to look for in a bra pad and others to avoid. When instructing mothers on bra pads:

1. Encourage the use of bra pads that are 100% cotton if the mother has sore nipples or a candida infection. Discourage use of pads with plastic liners and those made with synthetic fibers. Plastic liners and synthetic fibers trap surface moisture in near the skin and nipples, thus producing an environment that promotes nipple soreness. Pads made of 100% cotton allow air to circulate.

2. Encourage use of disposable pads made of pure paper (The First Years and Medela) or with polypropylene (Gerber Ultra Thin pad) or polyester/rayon layers that act as moisture barriers. In some products, the polyester/rayon layer is on the inside and not evident to the mother because it is not on the product label. Do not recommend pads with a plastic layer if a woman has sore nipples or a candida infection (Frantz, 1994). The capacity of the disposable pads ranges from three drops (The First Years and Medela) to 18 cc (Curity, Ameda/Egnell, Thrifty, and Leading Lady) (Frantz, 1994).

3. Encourage the use of white bra pads. Avoid pads that are colored using dyes. Some mothers may be sensitive to the dyes, and skin irritations may occur.

4. Instruct mothers to avoid using homemade pads that contain chemical residues (i.e., cutting up disposable diapers or sanitary napkins). Some mothers will have a skin-irritation reaction (Auerbach, 1987). Homemade pads of 100% cotton, dye-free material are acceptable.

5. Discuss the differences in the 22 brands of washable bra pads available. Twelve of these have a barrier of nylon or a plastic derivative (polypropylene, polyvinyl chloride, olefin) for moisture protection (Frantz, 1994). Use of pads with nylon or plastic derivative layers next to the breast is discouraged. Usually, bra pads have three layers: an inner layer next to the skin, usually made of cotton (preferred) but made of polyester in four brands (Medela, Leading Lady, Bobaby, and The Natural Choice Co.); a middle layer of absorbent filler containing rayon/polyester felt, flannel, plain felt, rayon, polyester, gauze, and cotton; and the outer layer made of a barrier fabric, nylon, or a plastic derivative, to protect the clothing from leakage (Frantz, 1994).

6. Explain the other considerations in choosing a washable bra pad: how much fluid it holds, laundering recommendations, size and shape of the pad, price, and availability. See *The Breastfeeding Product Guide* (Frantz, 1994) for an excellent overview of bra pads.

NURSING BRAS

When selecting a bra, the nursing mother should, if possible, choose one made of 100% cotton for increased comfort. If this is not possible, she should choose the one with the highest cotton content. She should try them on to determine the bra that offers the easiest access for her. Professionals usually recommend avoiding underwire bras because they may cause problems with plugged ducts and mastitis; but underwire styles are popular, and many women with large breasts prefer them. Bras containing plastic liners should be avoided; they trap surface moisture, which contributes to nipple tenderness and creates an excellent environment for candida infection. Bras with mid-cup seams may contribute to sore nipples and should also be avoided.

A tremendous variety of nursing bras are available in retail stores. In addition, many lactation consultants in private practice have expanded the retail component of their business to include the sale of nursing bras. Medela offers bra-fitting classes at various locations around the country. Leading Lady has a big selection of nursing bras, including bras designed to fit women who need larger sizes. Medela also has a free pumping attachment kit that secures a Medela breast pump kit to a Medela nursing bra for hands-free double breast pumping.

ENGORGEMENT BRAS

One bra currently on the market is designed specifically for the treatment of engorgement. It assists in treatment by providing coolant therapeutic measures. COOL-A-BRA is designed for use by women who experience engorgement during the early lactation period. The COOL-A-BRA provides relief for engorged breasts by allowing soft ice packs to be held in place over the breasts. It provides good support as well as easy convenience in removing or replacing the ice and feeding the infant. The COOL-A-BRA is available from the Nursing Mothers' Association of Australia. The association's address and phone number are provided in Section C of this chapter.

For a brief time, Medela, Inc., marketed an engorgement therapy bra that could be used for warm and cool therapy. This product is no longer available, however.

ICE FLOWERS/FLOWERPAK/INSTAHEAT PADS

Marmet and Shell (1981) successfully use "ice flowers" for assisting in the treatment of engorgement. Ice flowers are made by placing crushed ice in three small plastic sandwich bags and sealing each one. Each plastic bag is double-bagged by placing it inside another plastic bag. Again, each is sealed individually. Each bag of ice is considered a petal. The three petals are then tied together. A towel, cloth diaper, or handkerchief is placed on the breast and the ice flower applied, with each petal covering a different area of the breast. Ice flowers should never be placed directly on the breast (Marmet & Shell, 1981). Although this technique has not been documented in research studies, anecdotal reports indicate it has been widely and successfully used to reduce the swelling associated with engorgement.

FlowerPak (Ameda/Egnell) and InstaHeat pads (Medela) are two products designed to provide comfort and convenience for the breastfeeding mother needing hot or cold treatment for the breast. These products provide soothing warmth or coolness to the breast in a shape that fits comfortably on the breast.

CABBAGE COMPRESSES

The application of the clean, crisp, inner leaves of a cabbage as a compress has been successfully used for the treatment of engorgement and to suppress lactation. A substance, which has not yet been identified, is absorbed from the cabbage leaf through the mother's skin, resulting in decreased edema and improved milk flow. Extreme care and caution must be exercised when using the cabbage compress to treat engorgement; prolonged use may reduce the mother's milk supply. When the cabbage-compress technique is selected, it is important to assess the breasts prior to application and discuss the desired results with the lactating mother. Obtain a history, including any form of allergy or sensitivity to cabbage. If a sensitivity is present, the cabbage compress is contraindicated.

Thorough instructions must be given to the mother on the correct use of the cabbage compress. The inner leaves of the cabbage should be thoroughly washed and dried. The leaves are then placed in the bra, over the breast or breasts. Within two hours, or when the cabbage leaves have wilted, the leaves should be removed and the breasts inspected to see if the desired results have been obtained. In mothers experiencing engorgement, the cabbage-leaf therapy must be terminated as soon as the desired results are obtained—her milk supply can be greatly reduced if treatment continues too long. The time taken to produce desired results varies among individuals (Rosier, 1988). To suppress lactation, the cabbage-leaf therapy is continued for 24 to 48 hours, changing the leaves regularly (every 2–3 hours) until milk flow has stopped and the mother experiences no discomfort.

BREAST CREAMS AND OINTMENTS

Commercial creams and ointments for the breasts are not a necessary part of caring for the lactating breast. The methodical practice of breast cream or ointment application to the nipple, areola, or breasts should be discouraged (Lauwers & Woessner, 1989; Lawrence, 1992). Montgomery's tubercles, sebaceous glands of the areola and nipple areas, provide a natural bacteriostatic lubricant (called sebum) that helps protect the nipples when it is not removed or disturbed.

Encourage the mother to use her own hindmilk for a breast cream. At the end of a feeding, she should express a small amount of her breastmilk and gently pat it on the nipple and areola areas. She should then allow them to air dry. The hindmilk contains fats that are antibacterial and antiviral as well as other immunities that may help protect against infection (AAP, 1978; Lawrence, 1992). If the mother has candidiasis of the nipple area, she should not use her hindmilk for a breast cream because it provides the perfect environment for candida growth.

If a mother prefers to use a breast cream or ointment, she should be made aware of what to avoid and what may be best for her. The mother must choose a product that meets the high standards of being suitable and safe for the nursing mother's breasts and her breastfeeding infant. She should also be instructed in the proper use of the cream or ointment. The instructions should include making sure the nipple and areola areas are completely dry of any surface wetness before cream is applied and using only a small amount of the cream. The mother should avoid putting cream on the end of the nipple at the ductal openings—they can easily become plugged with repetitive applications of oily substances (Lawrence, 1992).

Occasionally a cream or ointment may cause a dermatitis of the skin where it is applied. If an irritation appears while any type of cream or ointment is being used on the breast, its use should be immediately discontinued. Lanolin products have a long history of causing allergic responses in a lanolin-sensitive population. The free-lanolin alcohol found naturally in lanolins has been identified as the allergic

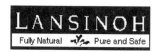

Figure 3B–1

Modified anhydrous lanolin—Lansinoh for breastfeeding mothers.

Source: Produced by Lansinoh Laboratories, Western Springs, IL. Reprinted with permission.

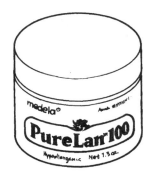

Figure 3B–2

Modified anhydrous lanolin—PureLan 100.

Source: Produced by Medela, Inc., McHenry, IL. PureLan is a registered trademark of Medela, Inc. Reprinted with permission.

component in lanolin. The greater the free-lanolin alcohol content, the greater the incidence of allergic response (Clark, 1975). Clinical trials indicate that at a level of 6.5% free-lanolin alcohol, 41% of a lanolin-sensitive population will continue to experience an allergic response. Even when the free-lanolin alcohol decreased to 3% and 2.2%, respectively, allergic responses were documented. Only when the level of free-lanolin alcohol was reduced to 1.5%, accompanied by an insignificant detergent content, were researchers unable to detect any allergic response among those who were considered sensitive to lanolin (Clark, Cronin, & Wilkinson, 1977).

Two widely used topicals containing lanolin are Lansinoh by Lansinoh Laboratories (Figure 3B–1) and PureLan 100 by Medela, Inc. (Figure 3B–2). Information supplied by the two companies follows: Lansinoh is an ultra-pure, medical grade of modified lanolin that is registered with the U.S. Food and Drug Administration (FDA) as an over-the-counter (OTC) drug. Lansinoh Laboratories guarantees their product never exceeds 1.5% free-lanolin alcohols and 0.05% detergent residue and contains less than 1 ppm total combined pesticide residue. These criteria meet the standards set by the United States Pharmacopeial Convention, Inc. (USP). Pure-Lan 100 contains less than 3% free-lanolin alcohols and less than 10 ppm of all combined pesticide residue. Medela has not published data regarding the detergent content of PureLan 100.

Creams and Ointments to Avoid

1. Those containing antibiotics, steroids, astringents, or bismuth subnitrate
   - Possibly harmful for infant and mother (Lawrence, 1992)
2. Those containing anesthetics
   - Milk-ejection reflex could be inhibited if nipples are numbed
   - May cause numbing of the infant's mouth, which could affect his or her sucking ability (Minchin, 1989)
3. Those containing alcohol
   - Drying to the nipple (Lauwers & Woessner, 1989; Minchin, 1989)
4. Those containing petroleum
   - Inhibits skin respiration, which may prolong nipple soreness (Lauwers & Woessner, 1989; Minchin, 1989)
5. Those containing peanut oil
   - Common allergen (Lauwers & Woessner, 1989)
6. Those containing crude grades of lanolin that do not meet the USP standards
   - USP standards are not more than 1 ppm of any individual pesticide and not more than a total of 3 ppm of all combined pesticide residues and a limit of 6% free-lanolin alcohol content (USP, 1992)
   - Women with sensitivities to wool may be affected by the impurities that are in some wool derivatives. Mothers have used lanolin to help soothe sore nipples for many years, but the free-lanolin alcohol content, combined with the detergent and pesticide residues, in lanolin compounds have caused a high percentage of allergic skin reactions. There are different grades and refinements of lanolin available for consumer purchase. They range from a pharmaceutical grade on the lower end of the scale, to a more pure medical grade on the upper end of the scale.
7. If manufacturer's instructions state to wash off prior to breastfeeding
   - If a product recommends it be washed off prior to breastfeeding, it is not intended for ingestion. Wiping or washing the cream off causes fric-

tion and irritation to already tender nipples and removes the natural lubrication (sebum) secreted by the Montgomery's tubercles.

8. Vitamin E
   - Use of vitamin E has been reported to increase serum vitamin E levels in infants (Marx et al., 1985)
   - Levels considered safe have not yet been determined.
   - Preparations with vitamin E are unsafe unless they are given by a professional for the treatment of a specific problem (Lawrence, 1989).

9. Aloe Vera
   - May cause diarrhea in the infant

Refer to Table 2B–2 in Chapter 2 of this module for specific questions to consider before selecting any topical for use on the breast.

NURSING STOOLS

A nursing stool is a small footstool made specifically to provide a comfortable way for the breastfeeding mother to elevate her feet while breastfeeding, thus elevating her lap and making her position more comfortable (see Figure 3B–3). The number one cause of sore nipples is improper positioning of the infant at breast. The nursing stool helps reduce some problems encountered when the infant is not brought to breast level for a feeding and, instead, the mother leans or bends over the infant. Use of the stool reduces stress on the mother's arms, shoulders, and lower back, thus avoiding strain and making the nursing experience more comfortable and enjoyable.

NURSING FASHIONS

The nursing mother's clothing need only do two things: allow easy access for discreet breastfeeding and provide the mother with comfortable clothing, promoting self-confidence and pride in her appearance. While nonspecialty clothing is more than appropriate for the lactating mother, some mothers prefer the ease and enjoy the looks that clothing made especially for the nursing mother may afford them.

Figure 3B–3

Typical nursing stool.

Source: Drawing courtesy of OrthoStools. Nursing Stool® is a registered trademark of OrthoStools, Inc., Payson, AZ. Reprinted with permission.

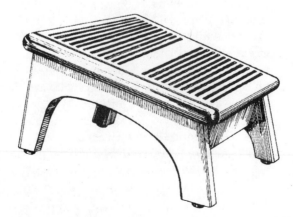

Clothing designed specifically for the breastfeeding mother may have hidden or disguised closures with Velcro, snaps, or zippers discreetly located in pleats, darts, seams, or under collars.

Patterns for the breastfeeding mother are available from Elizabeth Lee Designs and distributed by TLC Pillows. Pretty Private has nursing shawls to provide mothers who breastfeed in public a way to be discreet. The Lactation Institute (Encino, CA) offers a breastfeeding cape for use during consultations or for home use by mothers. MaMo Designs offers Natalis nursing scarves in two versions: a dressy white eyelet neckwrap and a casual blue chambray bib style.

Helpful Fashion Hints

1. Clothing made of cotton breathes easier. It is cooler in the summer months and warmer in the winter.
2. Light-colored clothing with prints helps disguise spots that may occur if the breastfeeding mother experiences leaking.
3. Two-piece outfits allow the breastfeeding mother easy access for breastfeeding. Outfits that button, zip, or fasten in the back are best avoided.
4. The openings in nightgowns/pajamas for the breastfeeding mother are oftentimes not large enough for comfortable and discreet access. The mother can easily enlarge the openings by cutting the seam of the opening a little further.

While many department stores and maternity shops offer some selections for the breastfeeding mother, shopping by catalog from companies in business specifically to sell breastfeeding fashions increases a mother's options. For further information, see the contacts/addresses located in Section C of this chapter.

NURSING PILLOWS

Several nursing pillows are now widely available—Nurse Mate by Four Dee Products; Boppy Pillow by Camp Kazoo, Ltd.; Loving Moms nursing pillow, TLC Baby Pillows, My Brest Friend by Zenoff Products—as well as pillows distributed by pump companies. During a breastfeeding session, the nursing mother's comfort and the infant's correct positioning at the breast are vitally important. The nursing pillow is a luxury, made specifically for the nursing mother. It assists her by comfortably supporting and resting her arm, as well as in bringing the infant up to breast level to achieve proper positioning.

BABY CARRIERS

There are many manufacturers of baby carriers. Medela has a Little Navigator, Parenting Concepts distributes the Sling-Ezee, and California Diversified Manufacturing distributes the Over the Shoulder Baby Holder. For those who sew, Elizabeth Lee Designs has a Bundle-N-Go Baby Carrier pattern. These carriers can be used by all mothers/babies but the slings are especially useful to breastfeeding mothers.

SCALES

Pediatric scales enable the mother or health-care provider to easily monitor the infant's intake by weighing him or her. They help maintain the breastfeeding relationship for at-risk infants and for premature infants with feeding difficulties. Scales help take the uncertainty out of intake when the infant's weight gain is critical. Medela introduced the BabyWeigh Scale to help monitor an infant's intake. It is available for sale; lease programs for professional use or rental for home use are also options.

The BabyWeigh Scale is portable, lightweight, and easy to operate. A prefeed weight and postfeed weight are taken; pushing one button calculates the breastmilk intake for that feeding session. It converts grams and pounds easily. Operation is fully automatic and accurate to 2 g for infants weighing less than 6000 g.

Medela also offers the BabyChecker scale for use with infants and toddlers weighing 6000 g or more. It does not have the ability to calculate the breastmilk intake based on pre- and postfeeding weights, but is a less expensive option for parents who would like to weigh their infants and toddlers at home.

Other pediatric electronic scales are also available. Health-O-Meter has one model (550 KL) that has a resolution of 10 g, is lightweight (8 lb) and can weigh infants and children up to a capacity of 44 lb (20 kg). Health Products, Inc., offers The Milky Weigh Scale. It is sensitive enough to calculate breastmilk intake and weighs up to 24 lb. The scale is accurate to 3 g for infants weighing 0 to 12 lb and 6 g for weights of 12 to 24 lb. The Home Health Digital Baby Scale has a weight capacity of 40 lb and weighs in increments of 0.5 ounces. It also measures in pounds or kilograms. It is available through Health Products, Inc.

Nursing Supplementer Devices

A nursing supplementer is a device that provides the infant with a supplement while the infant is nursing at the breast. The small, flexible tubing is attached to the breast and to a small plastic container/bag that contains the chosen supplement.

Nursing supplementers are invaluable in many circumstances. The device can help initiate a breastfeeding relationship that in some cases may not have been tried yet or rejuvenate one that may have failed. It allows the mother to receive the stimulation to her breasts that is necessary to support and increase her milk supply while providing a supplement to the infant. Nursing supplementer devices may also help avoid problems that may be encountered when supplementing with an artificial teat (nipple confusion) and enhance the bonding and intimacy of the breastfeeding relationship because the infant is supplemented at the breast for feedings.

Basic breastfeeding management should always be discussed and the nursing supplementer offered as an option when the situation is appropriate. Some mothers are intimidated by its appearance and see it as unnatural. Although using a nursing supplementer device may require more time in preparing, feeding, and cleaning up, it affords the mother an excellent option for supplementing her infant while avoiding artificial teats and increasing her own milk supply.

Human breastmilk is the number one supplement in almost all cases. If the mother chooses to supplement with her own milk, she should be assisted and instructed in the collection and storage of breastmilk. Some hospitals offer mothers access to a human milk bank. This can be discussed as an option.

Some mothers choose to use a manufactured formula as the supplement. If this is the case, the physician must recommend a formula and the mother be instructed in proper preparation and storage.

The physician should always be included in the care of the mother and infant using a nursing supplementer device. The infant needs to be monitored closely, including regular height, weight, and head circumference checks. The professional who has recommended its use to the mother should follow up frequently to make sure the infant's intake is adequate and the supplementer device is being used appropriately. It is also imperative that weaning from the device take place as soon as it is appropriate (Walker & Auerbach, 1993). Attention should also focus on maintaining the mother's milk supply when she is using a nursing supplementer device. Some lactation consultants report a decreased milk supply while these devices are being used. If this is the case, using an electric breast pump with the capacity to double-pump is indicated between feedings to maintain maternal milk supply.

The following list summarizes situations in which a nursing supplementer device may be appropriate (Auerbach, 1987; Walker & Auerbach, 1993):

1. Adoptive nursing
2. Relactation
3. Induced lactation
4. Failure-to-thrive infants
5. Infants with a weak or ineffective suck
6. Mothers with an inadequate milk supply

7. Premature infants
8. Infants who refuse to nurse
9. As a transition from bottle to breast
10. Infants who have a special physical need and require supplementation (i.e., those with Down syndrome, cleft lip, cleft palate, neurological impairments, cardiac problems)
11. Mothers with a history of breast surgery
12. Mothers who suffer from primary lactation insufficiency (Neifer & Seacat, 1985)
13. Mothers with severe nipple trauma
14. Mothers with flat or inverted nipples and infants that cannot latch on

AXI-CARE NURSING AID

The Axi-Care Nursing Aid (available only in the UK) nursing supplementer device is easy to assemble and has two sizes of tubing. Only one tube fits on the system at a time, so the tubing must be moved when the mother changes breasts. A stock clock is available for regulating the flow of supplement. A cleaning syringe is included.

LACT-AID

The Lact-Aid nursing trainer system is the first commercial nursing supplementer system ever made. It was developed in 1969 by Jimmie Lynne Avery and her husband, John Avery, as a way of nourishing their adopted child.

The Lact-Aid nursing training system contains a presterilized, 4-ounce (120 mL) plastic bag with one size of tubing. Only one tube fits on the system at a time, so the tubing must be moved when the mother changes breasts. Powdered formulas and meat-based formulas do not flow easily through the Lact-Aid device. A cleaning syringe is included (see Figure 3B–4).

Figure 3B–4
The Lact-Aid nursing trainer system.
Source: Drawing courtesy of Medical College of Georgia Hospital and Clinics, Augusta, GA. Reprinted with permission.

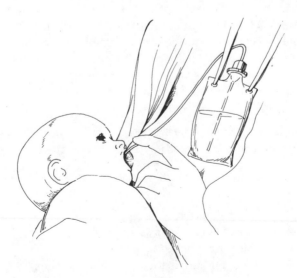

SUPPLEMENTAL NURSING SYSTEM

Medela produces the Supplemental Nursing System (SNS)—an open/vented system that contains an easy to assemble 6-ounce (180-ml) plastic bottle with tubing available in three sizes (small, medium, and large) for a variety of flow regulations. Two tubes fit on this system at once, which allows the mother to switch the infant from one breast to the other without having to move the tubing also. This system is easily cleaned; no cleaning syringe is necessary. The system's parts can be repeatedly autoclaved or boiled for long-term use. An instructional video tape is available.

STARTER SUPPLEMENTAL NURSING SYSTEM

Medela also offers an alternative to the large SNS—its Starter SNS. This is a smaller system and is more economical for short-term use. It consists of a one-way teat/valve that comes with a single, medium-sized tube and tubing clamp on an 80-cc plastic bottle. The Starter SNS can be purchased without the bottle for even lower cost—the user supplies the bottle. The parts of the Starter SNS can be autoclaved or boiled.

SUPPLY LINE

The Supply Line nursing supplementer device is available from the Nursing Mothers' Association of Australia (see contact information in Section C in this chapter). It contains an easy to assemble, 4-ounce (120-cc) bottle with pouch. One size tubing is available. Only one tube fits on the system at a time, so the tubing must be moved when the mother changes breasts. A cleaning syringe is included.

D-I-Y NURSING SUPPLEMENTER

The D-I-Y supplementer is available in the United Kingdom from Ann Buckley. It uses a regular-style bottle and artificial bottle teat. The tubing is inserted through the nipple into the bottle. The flow is regulated by the height at which the bottle is held.

Other Supplementing Techniques

FINGER FEEDING

Finger feeding is a method that can be used to supplement nourishment to an infant while teaching the infant to nurse more effectively and avoiding the use of bottles. A nursing supplementer device—syringe and gavage tube, or plastic dropper—may be used for finger feeding (Figures 3B–5 and 3B–6). Another alternative is to use the Hazelbaker Fingerfeeder. This device consists of a soft, pliable container for the supplement that is held in the palm of the hand and delivers milk to the baby through tubing taped to the finger. The supplement is provided by the device chosen, while the infant sucks on the caregiver's finger. The finger keeps the infant's tongue in place and dictates that the infant provide a correct suck in order to receive milk into his or her mouth.

Finger feeding is an excellent transitional tool and good for coaxing a reluctant nurser to the breast, but does not replace feeding at the mother's breast. Finger feeding may be used prior to offering the breast to the infant if he or she is having difficulty sucking (Barger & Bull, 1987). After a few minutes of finger feeding, the breast should be offered. If the infant is unable to properly latch on and suck at the breast after repeated attempts, the feeding may be completed by finger feeding.

Walker (1990) gives the following instructions on finger feeding:

1. Hands and nails should be clean. Fingernails should be clipped short. The finger is inserted nail side down, with the pad of the finger toward the infant's palate.

Figure 3B–5

Finger feeding using a gavage set.

Source: Drawing courtesy of Medical College of Georgia Hospital and Clinics, Augusta, GA. Reprinted with permission.

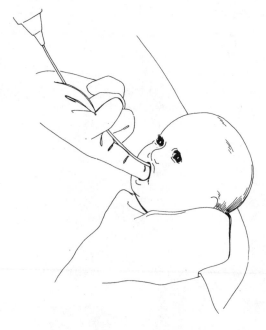

Figure 3B–6

Finger feeding using a periodontal syringe.

Source: Drawing courtesy of Medical College of Georgia Hospital and Clinics, Augusta, GA. Reprinted with permission.

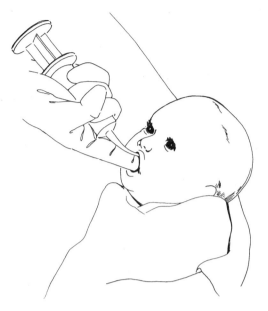

2. Position the infant so he or she is secure and the caregiver is comfortable. Two hands are required if a syringe or plastic dropper is used: take this into consideration when positioning the infant.
3. When a nursing supplementer device or gavage tube is used, the tubing can be taped to the pad of the small finger (or whichever digit is closest to the size of the mother's nipple). The tape should be placed far enough back on the digit so that the infant does not pull it into his or her mouth. The tubing may also be held rather than taped. The tubing size used depends on the condition of the infant and his or her ability to suck and swallow. Milk is removed only when the infant's suck is correct. This helps reinforce proper sucking, which may assist in a quicker and more effective transition to the breast.
4. If a plastic dropper is used, the caregiver should not squeeze or force the supplement into the infant's mouth—this could cause serious problems, such as gagging, aspiration, bradycardia, or reduced oxygenation.
5. The amount of supplement ingested should be recorded at each feeding session, along with any accomplishments or difficulties.

PERIODONTAL SYRINGE

The periodontal syringe is a tool used to provide supplemental nourishment to an infant while he or she is at the breast or finger feeding (see previous section on finger feeding and Figure 3B–6). The curved portion of the syringe is carefully supported on the breast or finger. The tip is inserted at the corner of the infant's mouth only after he or she is observed to be actively sucking and swallowing. The plunger should be pressed down extremely slowly to avoid complications, such as gagging, aspiration, bradycardia, or reduced oxygenation (Walker, 1990). Let the infant's ability to suck and swallow be your guide.

Figure 3B–7
Supplemental feeding device.

Source: Spangler, A (1995), *Breastfeeding, A Parent's Guide*, p. 65. Illustration by Abby Drue, Inc. Copyright © 1995 by Amy Kathryn Spangler. Reprinted with permission.

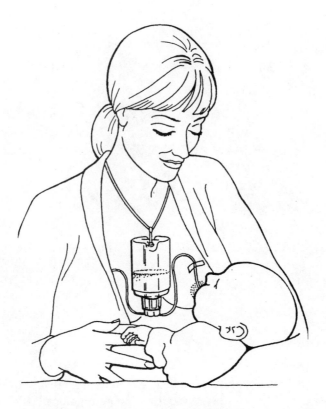

For one feeding session, one periodontal syringe may be filled and then refilled repeatedly as needed or multiple syringes may be filled and readied for use at the feeding. The supplement should not be stored in the syringe for longer than the time of a feeding.

The periodontal syringe should be cleaned after use; do not allow any supplement to dry on it. A syringe may be used multiple times; however, it may become difficult to use after a few times and should then be replaced. Periodontal syringes are inexpensive, so this should not present an obstacle.

CUP FEEDING

Cup feeding is another alternative method of supplementing the breastfed infant without the use of a bottle and artificial teat. The infant receives the benefits of the expressed breastmilk and avoids the possible confusion that may be introduced if given an artificial teat, thereby avoiding a multitude of possible difficulties. Cup feeding does not make the infant reluctant to suck at the breast. It may begin as early as immediately after birth if breastfeeding is unable to begin. If an infant can swallow, it is possible for him or her to drink from a cup for supplementation.

Specifics about Cup Feeding
1. An ordinary cup may be used. Cups with covers and spouts must be cleaned and sterilized as a bottle would be.

Note: Information on cup feeding is taken from the IBFAN Statement on Cups (IBFAN, 1993) and the Ameda/Egnell (1993) Baby Cup Feeding Instructions.

2. Wrap the infant securely in a blanket to help prevent his or her arms or hands from hitting the cup during a feeding.
3. The infant should be held in a comfortable position in the caregiver's arms and should be sitting in a supported, upright position on the caregiver's lap.
4. The cup should be held up to the infant's lips and tipped so the milk is just touching the lips. The cup should be tipped slowly so small amounts of milk are taken by the infant. Careful attention should be given not to tip the cup too far or too quickly so that large amounts pour into the infant's mouth.
5. Provide small sips of milk at a time, and offer short rest periods in-between—small, sick, or weak infants may need them. The infant will eventually set his or her own sipping rhythm.
6. The cup should remain in position at the infant's mouth during a feeding. Do not withdraw the cup if the infant stops drinking—the infant may be pausing for a rest. Let the infant set his or her own pace. (See Figure 3B–8.)

Ameda/Egnell produces a baby cup for simplifying cup feeding. Instruction sheets accompanying the cup are also available from Ameda/Egnell (Hollister, Inc.). Medela has designed a device for cup feeding called SoftCup. It provides caregivers with more control during cup feeding. The SoftCup is made of soft, pliable, pure silicone and is contoured for small mouths. It has a valve and self-refilling reservoir, so a steady supply of milk is available during feedings.

Figure 3B–8

Cup feeding an infant.

Source: King, FS (1992). *Helping Mothers to Breastfeed*, Revised Edition, p. 128. Nairobi, Kenya: AMREF. Reprinted with permission.

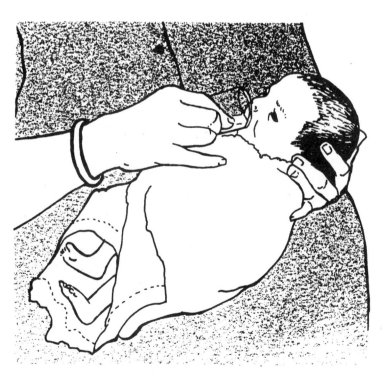

POST-TEST

For questions 1 to 6, choose the best answer from the following key:

A. True   B. False

1. Breast shells can cause plugged ducts and mastitis.

2. When choosing a bra pad, pads with designs and colored varieties are just as effective and appropriate as plain, white ones.

3. A nipple shield protects the nipple tissue from any possible damage.

4. A nursing bra with underwire support is most desirable because of the added support it provides the lactating breasts.

5. Vitamin E is one of the recommended topicals for the nursing mother's nipples.

6. The Haberman feeding device helps provide the infant with a supplement while the infant is sucking at the breast.

For questions 7 to 20, choose the best answer.

7. Ms. Smith is severely engorged at three weeks postpartum. Your management suggestions may include

    A. aggressive use of an electric breast pump every hour on a high-suction setting.
    B. use of ice flowers.
    C. use of an engorgement bra.
    D. Both A and C.
    E. Both B and C.

8. Appropriate topicals for the nursing mother's breasts include

    A. aloe vera.
    B. vitamin E.
    C. modified anhydrous lanolins meeting USP standards.
    D. All of the above.

9. A mother in her 37th week of pregnancy calls you for advice regarding her inverted nipples because she plans to breastfeed her infant. Your management suggestions include

    A. the use of breast shells. She should not begin wearing them until she is in her 40th week of pregnancy.
    B. using nipple shields as soon as possible.
    C. not setting her expectations too high because of her inverted nipples.
    D. None of the above.

10. Ms. Jones, who does not work outside the home, is in the process of choosing a bra pad. Of her choices, you advise her to choose

    A. the white pads with plastic leak-protection liners.
    B. the pink pads with the blue designs made of 100% cotton.
    C. the 100% cotton pads.
    D. None of the above.

11. If a plastic dropper is used for finger feeding, the caregiver should not force the supplement into the infant's mouth because that could cause

    A. bradycardia.
    B. reduced oxygenation.
    C. aspiration.
    D. All of the above.

12. Cup feeding as a method of supplementing the breastfed infant

    A. can begin when necessary, as soon as immediately following birth, if needed.
    B. should not begin until the infant is at least six days old.
    C. should not begin until the infant is at least six months old and beginning to sit unsupported.

13. Ms. Johnston has just purchased breast shells to begin wearing in her last six weeks of pregnancy because she has inverted nipples. Your instructions to her include

    A. gradually increasing the amount of time she wears the breast shells, beginning at 1 to 2 hours a day, slowly increasing the time until she reaches 6 to 10 hours a day.
    B. beginning to wear the breast shells around the clock because she is due soon.
    C. wearing the breast shells for 2 to 4 hours during her waking hours and all night while sleeping.
    D. wearing a very snug bra that holds the breast shells tightly against her breast. This will help correct the inversion.

14. The continuous use of a nipple shield decreases the amount of milk the infant receives

    A. by as much as 22% when a thick gum rubber nipple shield is used and as much as 58% when a thin silicone shield is used.
    B. by as much as 58% when a thick gum rubber nipple shield is used and as much as 22% when a thin silicone shield is used.
    C. The statement is untrue. When used correctly, the nipple shield will not affect the amount of milk the infant receives from his or her mother while breastfeeding.
    D. None of the above.

15. Possible problems associated with use of the nipple shield include

    A. ineffective sucking patterns.
    B. contributing to slow weight gain by the infant.
    C. potential for nipple and areola tissue damage.
    D. Both A and B.
    E. All of the above.

16. An alternative to using the nipple shield when the mother is having difficulty because of flat nipples is

    A. rolling and shaping the nipple prior to breastfeeding.
    B. pumping briefly prior to the breastfeeding session.
    C. wearing breast shells between breastfeeding sessions.
    D. All of the above.

17. When using a nursing supplementer device,

    A. the physician should always be included in the care of the mother and infant.
    B. the infant needs to be monitored closely, including regular length, head circumference, and weight checks.
    C. the professional who has recommended the device should follow up frequently to assure adequate intake by the infant and proper use of the device.
    D. All of the above.

18. Situations in which a nursing supplementer device may be appropriate include
    A. infants with a weak or ineffective suck.
    B. mothers who say "I'm not making enough milk. My baby wants to breast-feed all the time."
    C. adoptive nursing.
    D. Both A and C.
    E. All of the above.

19. When finger feeding,
    A. the amount of the supplement ingested should be recorded at each feeding, along with any accomplishments or difficulties.
    B. the amount of the supplement fed to the infant should equal 30 cc per pound of body weight.
    C. the finger helps keep the infant's tongue in place and dictates that the infant suck correctly in order to receive milk into his or her mouth.
    D. All of the above.
    E. Both A and C.

20. _____ is (are) not necessary for a mother to have a successful breastfeeding relationship.
    A. A nursing stool
    B. Dresses designed specifically for the breastfeeding mother
    C. A nursing pillow
    D. A breast pump
    E. All of the above.

SECTION C

Resources

Jan B. Simpson, RN, BSN, IBCLC

LEARNING OBJECTIVES

At the completion of this section, the learner will be able to do the following:

1. Locate breast pumps and other breastfeeding accessories that may aid the breastfeeding mother.

BRA PADS

AMH Distributors of Hawaii
P.O. Box 1334
Ewa, HI 96706
(The Ultimate nursing pad)

Australia-Bobaby Pty, Ltd.
Merrily, Merrily Enterprises
P.O. Box 456
Caringhah, NSW 2229
Australia
Phone: 02-524-0757
(Bobaby breast pads)

Avent: MacNeil Babycare Limited
5161 Thatcher Rd.
Downers Grove, IL 60515
Phone: 800-542-8368 / 708-769-1700
Fax: 708-769-0300
(Avent washable breast pads)

Bosom Buddies
P.O. Box 6138
Kingston, NY 12401
Phone: 914-338-2038
(Bosom Buddies bra pads)

Evenflo Products Company
771 N. Freedom St.
P.O. Box 1206
Ravena, OH 44266-1206
Phone: 800-356-2229 / 216-296-3465
Fax: 216-296-8588
(Natural Mother nursing pad)

Gerber Products Company
445 State St.
Fremont, MI 49413-0001
Phone: 800-443-7237 / 616-928-2000
Fax: 616-928-2723
(Ultra thin nursing pads;
Super-absorbent nursing pads)

Graham-Field, Inc.
Consumer Products Division
400 Rabro Dr. E.
Hauppauge, NY 11788-4226
Phone: 800-645-1023 / 516-582-5900
Fax: 516-582-5608
(Gentle Expressions washable
nursing pads)

Hollister, Inc.
2000 Hollister Dr.
Libertyville, IL 60048
Phone: 800-323-4060 / 847-680-1000
Fax: 847-680-1017
(Curity® disposable nursing pads)

Indisposables Cotton Diaper Company
1955 McLean Dr.
Vancouver, BC V5N 3J7
Canada
Phone: 800-663-1760 / 604-251-3422
Fax: 604-251-3410
(Indisposables™ nursing pads)

International Design/Manufacturing
305 Avenue G
Redondo Beach, CA 90277
Phone: 310-543-1899
(Comfy-Dri pads)

Johnson & Johnson Consumer Products, Inc.
199 Grandview Rd.
Skillman, NJ 08558-9418
Phone: 800-526-3967
Fax: 908-874-1138
(Johnson's nursing pads)

Kendall Futuro Company
1 Riverfront Pl.
Newport, KY 41071
Phone: 606-655-3400
(Curity® nursing pads)

Kiddie Products, Inc.
One Kiddie Dr.
Avon, MA 02322
Phone: 800-533-6708 / 508-588-1220
Fax: 508-583-9067
(The First Years disposable, form-fitting nursing pads)

Kidpower Unlimited, Inc.
70 Don Park Rd., Unit 16
Markham, Ontario L3R 1G4
Canada
(Baby Matey)

Leading Lady
24050 Commerce Park Rd.
Beachwood, OH 44122
Phone: 216-464-9066
Fax: 216-464-9365
(Leading Lady® nursing pads)

Marshall Baby Products
Division of Omron Health Care, Inc.
300 Lakeview Pkwy.
Vernon Hills, IL 60061
Phone: 800-922-2959 / 708-680-6206
Fax: 708-680-6269
(Comfort Plus washable breast pads)

Medela, Inc.
4610 Prime Pkwy.
P.O. Box 660
McHenry, IL 60051-0660
Phone: 800-435-8316
(washable and disposable bra pads)

Milk Diapers
P.O. Box 961
Camas, WA 98607
Phone: 800-929-0218 / 206-253-8374
(Milk Diapers nursing pads)

Motherhood Maternity Shops
390 N. Sepulveda Blvd., #3000
El Segundo, CA 90245
Phone: 310-364-1100
Fax: 310-335-0014
(Motherhood nursing pads)

The Natural Choice Company
1155 Chess Dr., Suite 105
Foster City, CA 94404
Phone: 800-528-8887 / 415-571-6606
Fax: 415-571-1948
(Natural Choice nursing pads)

Nu Angel
P.O. Box 030132
Tuscaloosa, AL 35403
(washable nursing pads)

Nursing Mother Breast Pads
Division of Amdox Company, Ltd.
P.O. Box 324
Brantford, Ontario N3T 5N3
Canada
Phone: 519-756-8722
(reusable breast pads)

Tamara Dee, Inc.
9057 Greenwood Ave. N.
Seattle, WA 98130
Phone: 206-784-7777
(Leite breast pads)

Thrifty Drugs
Baby Products Division
3424 Wilshire Blvd.
Los Angeles, CA 90005
Phone: 213-251-6000
(Thrifty disposable nursing pads)

TL Care Inc.
P.O. Box 77087
San Francisco, CA 94107
Phone: 415-626-3127
Fax: 415-626-2983
(TL Care washable nursing pads)

BREAST LEAKAGE SYSTEMS

Prolac, Inc.
P.O. Box 130
Skaneateles, NY 13152
Phone: 315-685-1955
Fax: 315-685-0447
(*blis* breast leakage inhibitor system)

BREAST PUMPS
Battery-Powered Breast Pumps

Evenflo Products Company
771 N. Freedom St.
P.O. Box 1206
Ravenna, OH 44266-1206
Phone: 800-356-2229 / 216-296-3465
(Evenflo Soft Touch Ultra)

Graham-Field, Inc.
400 Rabro Dr. E.
Hauppauge, NY 11788-4226
Phone: 800-645-1023 / 516-582-5900
Fax: 516-582-5608
(Gentle Expressions breast pump)

Hollister, Inc.
2000 Hollister Dr.
Libertyville, IL 60048
Phone: 800-323-4060 / 847-680-1000
Fax: 847-680-1017
(Ameda/Egnell Lact-B battery-powered
breast pump)

La Leche League International
1400 N. Meacham Rd.
P.O. Box 4079
Schaumburg, IL 60168-4079
Phone: 708-519-7730
Fax: 708-519-0035

Omron Healthcare, Inc.
300 Lakeview Pkwy.
Vernon Hills, IL 60061
Phone: 800-231-4030 / 847-680-6200
Fax: 847-680-6269
(Mag Mag battery-operated
breast pumps)

Pigeon Corp.
5-1, Tomlyame, Kanda
Chiyoda-Ku, Tokyo 101
Japan
Phone: 81-03-325 24111
Fax: 81-03-325 24029
(Pigeon Pump & Feed)

Manually Operated Breast Pumps

Cannon Babysafe, Ltd.
Lower Rd.
Glemsford, Suffolk
England CO10 7QS
(Avent manual breast pump)

Evenflo Products Company
771 N. Freedom St.
P.O. Box 1206
Ravenna, OH 44266-1206
Phone: 800-356-2229 / 216-296-3465
(Evenflo bulb manual breast pump)

Gerber Products Company
445 State St.
Fremont, MI 49413-0001
Phone: 800-443-7237 / 616-928-2000
Fax: 616-928-2723
(Precious Care manual breast pump)

Hollister, Inc.
2000 Hollister Dr.
Libertyville, IL 60048
Phone: 800-323-4060 / 847-680-1000
Fax: 847-680-1017
(Ameda/Egnell cylinder hand and one-hand
breast pumps)

International Design/Manufacturing, Inc.
305 Avenue G
Redondo Beach, CA 90277
Phone: 310-543-1899

Kids Corp. International
11500 S.W. 120th St.
Miami, FL 33176

La Leche League International
1400 N. Meacham Rd.
P.O. Box 4079
Schaumburg, IL 60168-4079
Phone: 708-519-7730
Fax: 708-519-0035

Lopuco, Ltd.
1615 Old Annapolis Rd.
Woodbine, MD 21797
(Loyd-B breast pump)

Lunas Enterprises
P.O. Box 2400
Sitka, AK 99835
(Ora'lac breast pump)

Medela, Inc.
4610 Prime Pkwy.
P.O. Box 660
McHenry, IL 60051-0660
Phone: 800-435-8316
(Manualelectric® breast pump)

Omron Healthcare, Inc.
300 Lakeview Pkwy.
Vernon Hills, IL 60061
Phone: 800-231-4030 / 847-680-6200
Fax: 847-680-6269
(Comfort Plus cylinder
breast pump)

Sassy, Inc.
1534 College S.E.
Grand Rapids, MI 49507
(Infa cylinder breast pump)

White River Corp.
Division of Natural Technologies, Inc.
924 C Calle Negocio
San Clemente, CA 92673
Phone: 800-824-6351 / 714-366-8960
Fax: 714-366-1664
(White River Natural Technologies
breast pump model 500)

Electric Breast Pumps

Bailey Medical Engineering
2216 Sunset Dr.
Los Osos, CA 93402
Phone: 800-413-3216 / 805-528-5781
(Nurture III semiautomatic breast pump)

Gerber Products Company
445 State St.
Fremont, MI 49413-0001
Phone: 800-443-7237 / 616-928-2000
Fax: 616-928-2723
(Precious Care electric breast pump)

Gomco Division
Allied Healthcare Products
1720 Sublette Ave.
St. Louis, MO 63110
Phone: 800-444-3954 / 314-771-2400
Fax: 800-477-7701
(Gomco® models #1118 and #218)

Graham-Field, Inc.
Consumer Products Division
400 Rabro Dr. E.
Hauppauge, NY 11788-4226
Phone: 800-645-1023 / 516-582-5900
Fax: 516-582-5608
(Gentle Expressions breast pump)

Hollister, Inc.
2000 Hollister Dr.
Libertyville, IL 60048
Phone: 800-323-4060 / 847-680-1000
Fax: 847-680-1017
(Ameda/Egnell SMB, Lact-E, Lact-E-lite, and Elite)

Medela, Inc.
4610 Prime Pkwy.
P.O. Box 660
McHenry, IL 60051-0660
Phone: 800-435-8316
(Classic 015, Lactina Select, Pump in Style, Mini-Electric, and Little Hearts™ breast pumps)

Schuco, Inc.
Allied Healthcare Products
1720 Sublette Ave.
St. Louis, MO 63110
Phone: 800-444-3954 / 314-771-2400
Fax: 800-477-7701
(Schuco® models #136 and #400)

White River Corp.
Division of Natural Technologies, Inc.
924 C Calle Negocio
San Clemente, CA 92673
Phone: 800-824-6351 / 714-366-8960
Fax: 714-366-1664
(White River Natural Technologies breast pumps 8900 and 9050)

BREAST SHELLS

Breastfeeding Support Consultants
228 Park Lane
Chalfont, PA 18914
Phone: 215-822-1281
Fax: 215-997-7879
(Sunburst breast shells)

CEA of Greater Philadelphia
127 Fayette St.
Conshohocken, PA 19428
Phone: 215-828-0131
(Comfi-Dri milk cups)

Hollister, Inc.
2000 Hollister Dr.
Libertyville, IL 60048
Phone: 800-323-4060 / 847-680-1000
Fax: 847-680-1017
(Ameda/Egnell breast shells)

La Leche League International
1400 N. Meacham Rd.
P.O. Box 4079
Schaumburg, IL 60168-4079
Phone: 708-519-7730
Fax: 708-519-0035
(breast shells)

Medela, Inc.
4610 Prime Pkwy.
P.O. Box 660
McHenry, IL 60051-0660
Phone: 800-435-8316

Nesty Company
34 Sunrise Ave.
Mill Valley, CA 94941
Phone: 415-388-3660
(milk cups)

Pharmics
1878 S. Redwood Rd.
Salt Lake City, UT 84104
Phone: 801-972-4138

CARRIERS FOR BABIES

California Diversified Manufacturing
919 Calle Amanecer, Suite L
San Clemente, CA 92673
Phone: 714-361-1089
(Over the Shoulder Baby Holder)

Elizabeth Lee Designs
P.O. Box 696
Bluebell, UT 84007
Phone: 801-454-3350
Fax: 801-454-3450
e-mail: eldesign@uwin.com
(Bundle-N-Go baby carrier pattern)

Medela, Inc.
4610 Prime Pkwy.
P.O. Box 660
McHenry, IL 60051-0660
Phone: 800-435-8316
(Little Navigator™)

Parenting Concepts
P.O. Box 1437
Lake Arrowhead, CA 92352
Phone: 909-337-1499
(Sling Ezee)

ENGORGEMENT THERAPY PRODUCTS

Medela, Inc.
4610 Prime Pkwy.
P.O. Box 660
McHenry, IL 60051-0660
Phone: 800-435-8316
(InstaHeat™ pads)

Nursing Mothers' Association of Australia
P.O. Box 231
Nunawading, Victoria 3131
Australia
Phone: 613-877-5011
(Cool-A-Bra engorgement bra)

FINGERFEEDING DEVICES

Medela, Inc.
4610 Prime Pkwy.
P.O. Box 660
McHenry, IL 60051-0660
Phone: 800-435-8316
(Hazelbaker fingerfeeder)

FREEZER BAGS FOR BREASTMILK

Breastfeeding Support Network, Inc.
2028 W. 9th Ave.
Oshkosh, WI 54901
Phone: 920-231-1611 / 888-MOMS BAGS
Fax: 920-231-1697
(Mother's Milk Storage Bags®)

Hollister, Inc.
2000 Hollister Dr.
Libertyville, IL 60048
Phone: 800-323-4060 / 847-680-1000
Fax: 847-680-1017
(Ameda/Egnell Mother's Milk freezer bags)

La Leche League International
1400 N. Meacham Rd.
P.O. Box 4079
Schaumburg, IL 60168-4079
Phone: 708-519-7730
Fax: 708-519-0035

Medela, Inc.
4610 Prime Pkwy.
P.O. Box 660
McHenry, IL 60051-0660
Phone: 800-435-8316
(Medela breastmilk bags)

FUNNELS FOR MANUAL EXPRESSION

La Leche League International
1400 N. Meacham Rd.
P.O. Box 4079
Schaumburg, IL 60168-4079
Phone: 708-519-7730
Fax: 708-519-0035

Medela, Inc.
4610 Prime Pkwy., P.O. Box 660
McHenry, IL 60051-0660
Phone: 800-435-8316

INFANT FEEDING CUPS

Foley Development, Inc.
6232 Paradise Trail
Carp Lake, MI 49718
Phone: 888-INFANT-8 / 616-537-3030
(Infant Input cup feeder)

Hollister, Inc.
2000 Hollister Dr.
Libertyville, IL 60048
Phone: 800-323-4060 / 847-680-1000
Fax: 847-680-1017
(Ameda/Egnell baby cup)

Medela, Inc.
4610 Prime Pkwy.
P.O. Box 660
McHenry, IL 60051-0660
Phone: 800-435-8316
(SoftCup infant feeding cup)

INSULATED CARRIERS FOR EXPRESSED MILK

Bosom Buddies
P.O. Box 6138
Kingston, NY 12401
Phone: 914-338-2038

Lact-Aid International, Inc.
P.O. Box 1066
Athens, TN 37303

MODIFIED LANOLIN

Hollister, Inc.
2000 Hollister Dr.
Libertyville, IL 60048
Phone: 800-323-4060 / 847-680-1000
Fax: 847-680-1017
(Lansinoh®)

La Leche League International
1400 N. Meacham Rd.
P.O. Box 4079
Schaumburg, IL 60168-4079
Phone: 708-519-7730
Fax: 708-519-0035
(Lansinoh)

Lansinoh Laboratories, Inc.
1670 Oak Ridge Tpke.
Oak Ridge, TN 37830
Phone: 800-292-4794
(Lansinoh®)

Medela, Inc.
4610 Prime Pkwy.
P.O. Box 660
McHenry, IL 60051-0660
Phone: 800-435-8316
(PureLan™ 100)

NIPPLE SHIELDS

Cannon Babysafe, Ltd.
Lower Rd.
Glemsford, Suffolk CO10 7QS
England

Hollister, Inc.
2000 Hollister Dr.
Libertyville, IL 60048
Phone: 800-323-4060 / 847-680-1000
Fax: 847-680-1017
(Ameda/Egnell nipple shield)

Medela, Inc.
4610 Prime Pkwy.
P.O. Box 660
McHenry, IL 60051-0660
Phone: 800-435-8316

NURSING BRAS

Bosom Buddies
P.O. Box 6138
Kingston, NY 12401
Phone: 914-338-2038

Bravado Designs
68 Broadview Ave.
Toronto, Ontario M4M 2E6
Canada
Phone: 416-466-8652

CI Medical, Inc.
6600 W. Rogers Cir.
Boca Raton, FL 33487
Phone: 800-889-8421 / 407-241-5663
Fax: 407-241-5646
(Maturna™ Bra System)

Decent Exposures
2202 N.E. 115, Dept. 405
Seattle, WA 98125

Delices for Nursing Mothers
4131 Madrona Way N.
Tacoma, WA 98407

Leading Lady
24050 Commerce Park Rd.
Beachwood, OH 44122
Phone: 216-464-9066
Fax: 216-464-9365
(several softcup and underwire styles)

Medela, Inc.
4610 Prime Pkwy.
P.O. Box 660
McHenry, IL 60051-0660
Phone: 800-435-8316
(softcup and underwire styles; Pumping Free™
attachment kit; SoftSupport bra strap pads)

Playtex Apparel, Inc.
Playtex Park
P.O. Box 631
Dover, DE 19903

NURSING FASHIONS

**Association for Breastfeeding
Fashions**
P.O. Box 4378
Sunland, CA 91041

Diana Designs
160 River Forest Dr.
Fayetteville, GA 30214
(Baby 'n' Me nursing bib)

Elizabeth Lee Designs
P.O. Box 696
Bluebell, UT 84007
Phone: 801-454-3350
Fax: 801-454-3450
eldesign@uwin.com

The 4th Trimester
Professional Bldg. North
2700 Hospital Dr., #470
N. Kansas City, MO 64116

The Lactation Institute
16430 Ventura Blvd.
Suite 303
Encino, CA 91436-2125
(breastfeeding cape)

MaMo Designs
133 Kirk Crossing
Decatur, GA 30030
Phone: 404-377-4728
(Natali™ breastfeeding
neckwrap and bib)

Medela, Inc.
4610 Prime Pkwy.
P.O. Box 660
McHenry, IL 60051-0660
Phone: 800-435-8316
(Looking Good Gown™)

Motherwear
P.O. Box 114NC
Northampton, MA 01061-0114

Precious Image Creations
P.O. Box 1559
Loganville, GA 30249

Pretty/Private™
943 N. Orlando
Mesa, AZ 85205
Phone: 800-795-8170
(nursing shawl)

Simply Delicious Nursingwear™
P.O. Box 5191
San Clemente, CA 92674
Phone: 800-637-9426 / 714-361-1089
(clothing)

NURSING PILLOWS

Baby Care
P.O. Box 5620
San Mateo, CA 94402
Phone: 415-572-2689
(nursing and baby feeding pillow)

Body Therapeutics Inc.
12501 Philadelphia St., #102
Whittier, CA 90601
Phone: 301-945-8141
Fax: 301-995-7759
(Pregnancy Wedge™)

Camp Kazoo, Ltd.
602 Park Point Dr., #150
Golden, CO 80401
Phone: 303-526-2626
Fax: 303-526-5470
(Boppy Pillow)

Judy Kreissman
348 Florence Ave.
Sebastopol, CA 95472
707-823-8260
(The Nursing Wedge®)

Loving Moms
P.O. Box 147
Skokie, IL 60076-0147
(Loving Moms nursing pillow)

Medela, Inc.
4610 Prime Pkwy.
P.O. Box 660
McHenry, IL 60051-0660
Phone: 800-435-8316
(Medela's Nursing Pillow)

My B*rest* Friend
Zenoff Products, LLC
157 Ovell Ave.
Mill Valley, CA 94941
Phone: 800-555-5522 / 415-383-1450
Fax: 415-383-3779

Noel Joanna, Inc.
22942 Arroyo Vista
Rancho Santa Margarita, CA 92688
Phone: 714-858-9717
Fax: 714-858-9686
(NoJo® nursing pillow)

TLC Baby Pillows
P.O. Box 25217
Oklahoma City, OK 73125
Phone: 405-677-3112
(TLC Baby Pillows)

Two by Two
A Division of Four Dee Products
13312 Redfish Lane, #104
Stafford, TX 77477
Phone: 800-526-2594 / 281-261-5510
Fax: 281-261-5442
e-mail: 4dee@ghgcorp.com
(Nurse Mate nursing pillow)

NURSING STOOLS

Hollister, Inc.
2000 Hollister Dr.
Libertyville, IL 60048
Phone: 800-323-4060 / 847-680-1000
Fax: 847-680-1017
(Mom's Favorite Footrest)

Medela, Inc.
4610 Prime Pkwy.
P.O. Box 660
McHenry, IL 60051-0660
Phone: 800-435-8316

OrthoStools, Inc.
608 N. Colcord Ave.
Payson, AZ 85541
Phone: 520-472-9022

NURSING SUPPLEMENTER DEVICES

Colgate Medical Ltd.
Fairacres Estate, Dedword Rd.
Windsor, Berks SL4 4LE
United Kingdom
(Axi-Care Nursing Supplementer)

D-I-Y Nursing Supplementer
Ann Buckley
14 Brookway, Grasscroft, Oldham
Lancashire
United Kingdom

Lact-Aid International, Inc.
P.O. Box 1066
Athens, TN 37303
(Lact-Aid nursing trainer)

La Leche League International
1400 N. Meacham Rd.
P.O. Box 4079
Schaumburg, IL 60168-4079
Phone: 708-519-7730
Fax: 708-519-0035

Medela, Inc.
4610 Prime Pkwy.
P.O. Box 660
McHenry, IL 60051-0660
Phone: 800-435-8316
(Supplemental Nursing System (SNS); Starter SNS;
Hazelbaker Finger-feeder)

Nursing Mothers Association of Australia
Merrily, Merrily Enterprises
P.O. Box 231
Nunawading
3131 Victoria, Australia
Phone: 61-3877-5011
Fax: 61-3894-3270
(Supply line)

SCALES

Health Products Incorporated
460 Lynden Dr.
Highland Heights, OH 44143-1565
Phone: 800-451-3890
Fax: 216-461-9659
(The Milky Weigh Baby Scale and Home Health
Digital Baby Scale)

Medela, Inc.
4610 Prime Pkwy.
P.O. Box 660
McHenry, IL 60051-0660
Phone: 800-435-8316
(BabyWeigh and BabyChecker scales)

References

Alexander, JM, Grant, AM, Campbell, MJ (1993). Randomized control trial of breast shells and Hoffman's exercises for inverted and non-protractile nipples. *Br Med J*, 304:1030-32.

Amatayakul, K, Vutyavanich, T, Tanthayaphinant, O, Tovanabutra, S, Yupadee, Y, Drewett, RF (1987). Serum prolactin and cortisol levels after sucking for varying periods of time and the effect of a nipple shield. *Acta Obstet Gynecol Scand*, 66:47-51.

Ameda/Egnell, Inc. (1993). *Instructions for the Ameda/Egnell Baby Cup*. Cary, IL: Ameda/Egnell.

American Academy of Pediatrics (AAP), Committee on Nutrition, and Canadian Paediatric Society (CPS), Nutrition Committee (1978). Breastfeeding: A commentary in celebration of the international year of the child. *Pediatrics*, 62, 591-601.

Arnold, LD (1993a). Guidelines for the establishment and operation of human milk bank. In: Riordan, J, Auerbach, K (eds.), *Breastfeeding and Human Lactation*, Appendix 22-1, pp. 613-618. Boston: Jones and Bartlett.

Arnold, LD (1993b). Issues in Human Milk Banking. In: Riordan, J, Auerbach, K (eds.), *Breastfeeding and Human Lactation*, pp. 597-611. Boston: Jones and Bartlett.

Arnold, LD, Tully, MR (1991). *Guidelines for the Establishment and Operation of a Human Milk Bank*. West Hartford, CT: Human Milk Bank Association of North America.

Auerbach, KG (1987). *Breastfeeding Techniques and Devices*. LLLI Lactation Consultant Series, Unit 17. Garden City Park, NY: Avery Publishing Group.

Auerbach, KG (1990). The effect of nipple shields on maternal milk volume. *JOGNN*, 19:419-27.

Barger, J, Bull, P (1987). A comparison of the bacterial composition of breastmilk stored at room temperature and stored in the refrigerator. *Int J Child Educ*, 2:29-30.

Clark, EW, Cronin, E, Wilkinson, DS (1977). Lanolin with reduced sensitizing potential. *Contact Dermatitis*, 3:69-74.

Frantz, KB (1994). *Breastfeeding Product Guide*. Sunland, CA: Geddes Productions.

Garrett, A, Ashworth, M (1996). Nipple shields: Insight from two experts. *Medela Rental Roundup*, 13(4):6-7.

Garza, C, Hopkinson, J, Schanler, RJ (1986). Human milk banking. In: Howell, RR, Morriss, RH, Pickering, LH (Eds.), *Human Milk in Infant Nutrition and Health*, pp. 225-55. Springfield, IL: Charles C. Thomas.

Goldblum, RM, Garza, C, Johnson, CA, Goldman, AS, Nichols, BL (1981). Human milk banking I: Effects of container upon immunologic factors in mature milk. *Nutr Res*, 1:449-59.

Hamosh, M (1996). Breastfeeding and the working mother: Effect of time and temperature of short-term storage on proteolysis, lipolysis, and bacterial growth in milk. *Pediatrics* 97(4):492-98.

Hopkinson, J, Garza, C, Asquith, MT (1990). Human milk storage in glass containers (letter). *J Hum Lact*, 6:104-5.

Hopkinson, JM, Schanler, R, Garza, C (1988). Milk production by mothers of premature infants. *Pediatrics*, 81:815-20.

International Baby Food Action Network (IBFAN) (1993). *IBFAN Statement on Cups*. Nairobi, Kenya: IBFAN-Africa.

Jackson, DA, Woolridge, MW, Imong, SM, McLeod, CN, Yutabootr, Y, Wongsawat, L, Amatayakul, K, Baum, JD (1987). The automatic sampling shield: A device for sampling sucked breastmilk. *Early Hum Dev*, 15:295-306.

King, FS (1992). *Helping Mothers to Breastfeed*. Nairobi, Kenya: African Medical and Research Foundation.

Marmet, C (1988). Manual Expression of Breastmilk—Marmet Technique. Encino, CA: The Lactation Institute.

Marmet, C, Shell, E (1981). Lactation Specialist Reference Material. Unpublished. Encino, CA: The Lactation Institute.

Marmet, C, Shell, E (1987). Lactation Institute Forms: A Guide to Lactation Consultant Charting. Encino, CA: The Lactation Institute.

Minchin, MK (1989). *Breastfeeding Matters: What We Need to Know about Infant Feeding.* Victoria, Australia: Alma Publications and George Allen and Unwin.

Neifert, MR, Seacat, JM (1985). Milk yield and prolactin rise with simultaneous breast pumping. Paper presented at the Ambulatory Pediatric Association, Washington, DC, May 7-10.

Nwankwo, M (1988). Bacterial growth in expressed breastmilk. *Ann Trop Pediatr,* 8:92-95.

Pardou, A (1994). Human milk banking: Influence of storage processes and of bacterial contamination on some milk constituents. *Biol Neonate,* 65:302-9.

Paxson, CL, Cress, CC (1979). Survival of human milk leukocytes, *J Pediatrics,* 94:61.

Pittard, WB (1985). Bacteriostatic qualities of human milk. *J Pediatr,* 107:240-43.

Pittard, WB, Geddis, KM, Brown, S (1991). Bacterial contamination of human milk: Container type and method of expression. *Am J Perinatol,* 8:25-27.

Rosier, W (1988). Cool cabbage compresses. *Breastfeeding Rev,* May:28-31.

Smith, MK (1992). Breastfeeding answers: Pumping and storing breastmilk. Cary, IL: Ameda/Egnell.

Sosa, R, Barness, L (1987). Bacterial growth in refrigerated human milk. *Am J Dis Child,* 141:111-12.

Spangler, A (1995). *Breastfeeding, A Parent's Guide,* p. 65. Atlanta, GA.

United States Pharmacopeial Convention, Inc. (USP) (1992). USP Pharmacy Board Bulletin: USP Changes Anhydrous Lanolin Monograph and Adds Modified Lanolin Monograph. USP: Rockville, MD.

Walker, M (1990). *Breastfeeding Premature Babies.* LLLI Lactation Consultant Series, Unit 14. Garden City Park, NY: Avery Publishing Group.

Walker, M, Auerbach, KG (1993). Breast Pumps and Other Technologies. In: Riordan, J, Auerbach, KG (eds.), *Breastfeeding and Human Lactation.* Boston: Jones and Bartlett.

Williamson, M, Murti, P (1996). Effects of storage, time, temperature and composition of containers on biologic components of human milk. *J Hum Lact,* 12(1):31-35.

Woolridge, MW, Baum, JD, Drewett, RF (1980). Effect of a traditional and of a new nipple shield on sucking patterns and milk flow. *Early Hum Dev,* 4:357-64.

ADDITIONAL READINGS

Ameda/Egnell, Inc. *Flexishield Nipple Stimulator.* Cary, IL: Ameda/Egnell.

Ameda/Egnell, Inc. *Mother's Touch One-Hand Breast Pump.* Cary, IL: Ameda/Egnell.

Ameda/Egnell, Inc. *Ameda/Egnell Breast Shell and Dual Pad System.* Cary, IL: Ameda/Egnell.

American Academy of Pediatrics, Committee on Nutrition (1980). Human milk banking. *Pediatrics,* 65:854-857.

Asquith, MT, Pedrotti, PW, Stevenson, DK, Sunshine, P (1987). Clinical uses, collection and banking of human milk. *Clin Perinatol,* 14:173-85.

Avent: MacNeil Babycare Limited. *Avent Naturally.* Downers Grove, IL: MacNeil Babycare Limited.

Bailey Medical Engineering. *Nurture III Electric Breast Pump.* Los Osos, CA: Bailey Medical Engineering.

Balmer, SE, Wharton, BA (1992). Human milk banking at Sorrento Maternity Hospital, Birmingham. *Arch Dis Child,* 67:556-59.

Bocar, DL (1993). *Breastfeeding Educator Program.* Oklahoma City: Lactation Consultant Services.

Borman, LL, Coates, MM (1990). Human milk banking. In: *The Lactation Consultant's Topical Review and Bibliography of the Literature on Breastfeeding,* pp. 135-38. Franklin Park, IL: La Leche League International.

Canadian Paediatric Society Nutrition Committee (1985). Statement on human milk banking. *Can Med Assoc J,* 132:750-52.

Clark, EW (1975). Estimate of the general incidence of specific lanolin allergy. *J Soc Cosmet Chem,* 26:323-25.

Davis, MK (1990). The role of human milk in human immunodeficiency virus infection. In: Atkinson, SA, Hanson, LA, Chandra, RK (eds.), *Breastfeeding, Nutrition, Infection and Infant Growth in Developed and Emerging Countries,* pp. 151-60. Human Lactation 4. St. John's, Newfoundland, Canada: ARTS Biomedical Publishers.

DeNicola, M (1986). One case of nipple shield addiction. *J Hum Lact,* 2:28-29.

Garza, C (1990). Banked human milk for very low birth weight infants. In: Atkinson, SA, Hanson, LA, Chandra, RK (eds.), *Breastfeeding, Nutrition, Infection and Infant Growth in Developed and Emerging Countries,* pp. 25-36. Human Lactation 4. St. John's, Newfoundland, Canada: ARTS Biomedical Publishers.

Garza, C, Nichols, BL (1984). Studies of human milk relevant to milk banking. *J Amer Coll Nutr,* 3:123-29.

Graham-Field, Inc. *Gentle Expressions: The Complete Line of Nursing Products.* Hauppauge, NY: Graham-Field, Inc., Consumer Product Division.

Isaacs, CE, Thormar, H (1990). Human milk lipids inactivate enveloped viruses. In: Atkinson, SA, Hanson, LA, Chandra, RK (eds.), *Breastfeeding, Nutrition, Infection and Infant Growth in Developed and Emerging Countries,* pp. 161-74. Human Lacation 4. St. John's, Newfoundland, Canada: ARTS Biomedical Publishers.

La Leche League International (1990). Human milk storage information. *Leaven,* Sept.-Oct., p. 69.

Lact-Aid International, Inc. *If it doesn't say—Lact-Aid.* Athens, TN: Lact-Aid.

Lauwers, J, Woessner, C (1989). *Counseling the Nursing Mother.* Garden City Park, NY: Avery Publishing.

Law, BJ, Urias, BA, Lertzman, Robson, D, Romance, L (1989). Is ingestion of milk-associated bacteria by premature infants fed raw human milk controlled by routine bacteriologic screening? *J Clin Microbiol,* 27:1560-66.

Lawrence, RA (1992). *Breastfeeding: A Guide for the Medical Profession.* St. Louis: C.V. Mosby.

Marmet, C, Shell, E (1988). Instruments used in breast-feeding management. In: Jelliffe, D, Jelliffe, EFP. *Programmes to Promote Breastfeeding.* Oxford: Oxford University Press.

Marshall Baby Products. *Making Successful Breast-feeding Easier.* Vernon Hills, IL: Marshall Baby Products.

Marx, CM, Izquierdo, A, Driscoll, JW, Murray, MA, Epstein, MF (1985). Vitamin E concentrations in serum of newborn infants after topical use of vitamin E by nursing mothers. *Am J Obstet Gynecol,* 152: 668-70.

McDougal, JS, Martin, LS, Cort, SP, Mozen, M, Heldebrant, CM, Evatt, BL (1985). Thermal inactivation of the acquired immunodeficiency virus, human T lymphotropic virus-III/lymphadenopathy-associated virus with special reference to antihemophilic factor. *J Clin Invest,* 76:875-77.

Medela, Inc. (1992). *Breastfeeding Information Guide: Breastfeeding Tips and Products.* McHenry, IL: Medela.

Medela, Inc. (1997). *Medela Breastfeeding Products.* McHenry, IL: Medela.

Medela, Inc. (1997). *Medela Hospital Catalogue.* McHenry, IL: Medela.

Michaelsen, KF, Skafte, L, Badsberg, JH, Jorgensen, M (1990). Variation in macronutrients in human bank milk: Influencing factors and implications for human milk banking. *J Pediatr Gastroent Nutr,* 11:229-39.

Narayanan, I (1982). Human milk in the developing world: To bank or not to bank? *Ind Pediatr,* 19:395-99.

Narayanan, I, Prakesh, K, Gujral, VV (1982). Management of expressed human milk in a developing country. Experiences and practical guidelines. *J Trop Pediatr,* 28:25-28.

Neifert, MR, Seacat, JM (1988). Practical aspects of breast-feeding the premature infant. *Perinatol/Neonatol,* 12:24-30.

Neville, MC, Neifert, MR (1983*). Lactation: Physiology, Nutrition, and Breastfeeding.* New York: Plenum Press.

Rangecroft, L, de San Lazaro, C, Scott, JES (1978). A comparison of the feeding of the postoperative newborn with banked breast-milk or cow's-milk feeds. *J Pediatr Surg,* 13:11-12.

Rees, D (1977). Juice-jar breast pump. *Keep Abreast J,* 2:225.

Riordan, J (1991). *A Practical Guide to Breastfeeding.* St. Louis: C.V. Mosby.

Williams, AF, Baum, JD (eds) (1984). *Human milk banking.* Nestle Nutrition Workshop Series. New York: Raven Press.

Williamson, S, Hewitt, JH, Finucane, E , Gamsu, HR (1978). Organization of bank of raw and pasteurized human milk for neonatal intensive care. *Brit Med J,* 1:393-96.

Pre- and Post-Test Answer Keys

Preparing to Breastfeed

Pre-Test	Post-Test
1. D	1. A
2. C	2. D
3. C	3. B
4. C	4. B
5. E	5. D
6. A	6. E
7. D	7. A
8. C	8. C
9. B	9. B
10. B	10. B
11. B	11. A
12. A	12. C
13. B	13. D
14. A	14. B
15. C	15. B
16. D	16. A
17. A	17. B
18. A	18. B
19. D	19. B
20. D	20. B

Feeding at the Breast

Pre-Test	Post-Test
1. B	1. B
2. A	2. D
3. C	3. B
4. A	4. C
5. B	5. A
6. D	6. C
7. B	7. A
8. C	8. B
9. A	9. D
10. D	10. D
11. D	11. C
12. C	12. B
13. C	13. C
14. A	14. B
15. C	15. A
16. B	16. D
17. C	17. D
18. A	18. B
19. D	19. D
20. C	20. C

Breastfeeding Assessment

Pre-Test	Post-Test
1. B	1. C
2. A	2. A
3. C	3. B
4. C	4. D
5. C	5. D
6. A	6. C
7. B	7. B
8. E	8. D
9. D	9. B
10. A	10. C
11. D	11. D
12. B	12. A
13. C	13. C
14. C	14. C
15. C	15. B
16. B	16. D
17. C	17. A
18. D	18. D
19. D	19. B
20. C	20. C

Areolar and Nipple Tissue Structural Elements and Wound Healing

Pre-Test	Post-Test
1. D	1. A
2. B	2. B
3. C	3. B
4. A	4. D
5. E	5. C
6. D	6. B
7. C	7. B
8. C	8. A
9. D	9. C
10. A	10. C
11. C	11. A
12. B	12. A
13. A	13. A
14. C	14. B
15. A	15. A
16. B	16. A
17. A	17. B
18. B	18. A
19. C	19. A
20. D	20. B

Nipple Soreness

Pre-Test	Post-Test
1. C	1. B
2. C	2. A
3. B	3. B
4. C	4. B
5. D	5. B
6. D	6. A
7. A	7. D
8. B	8. C
9. A	9. C
10. D	10. A
11. C	11. B
12. A	12. B
13. A	13. A
14. B	14. A
15. B	15. B
16. B	16. B
17. B	17. B
18. B	18. A
19. B	19. A
20. A	20. B

Breast-Related Problems

Pre-Test	Post-Test
1. A	1. E
2. D	2. E
3. D	3. D
4. A	4. B
5. C	5. C
6. A	6. A
7. D	7. B
8. D	8. A
9. E	9. B
10. A	10. A
11. C	11. A
12. D	12. A
13. B	13. B
14. D	14. C
15. E	15. A
16. A	16. D
17. B	17. B
18. A	18. D
19. A	19. A
20. A	20. C

Infant-Related Problems

Pre-Test	Post-Test
1. D	1. C
2. E	2. D
3. B	3. B
4. D	4. E
5. D	5. A
6. B	6. B
7. E	7. B
8. E	8. D
9. A	9. D
10. A	10. B
11. A	11. D
12. B	12. A
13. D	13. C
14. B	14. A
15. B	15. A
16. A	16. B
17. B	17. A
18. A	18. B
19. B	19. A
20. A	20. B

Expression, Collection, and Storage of Breastmilk

Pre-Test	Post-Test
1. D	1. C
2. C	2. C
3. B	3. B
4. C	4. C
5. C	5. A
6. C	6. B
7. D	7. C
8. E	8. D
9. A	9. A
10. A	10. C
11. A	11. B
12. C	12. B
13. A	13. B
14. D	14. B
15. E	15. B
16. B	16. C
17. B	17. B
18. B	18. B
19. A	19. E
20. B	20. B

Breastfeeding Accessories, Devices, and Supplemental Techniques

Pre-Test	Post-Test
1. E	1. A
2. A	2. B
3. B	3. B
4. E	4. B
5. D	5. B
6. D	6. B
7. E	7. E
8. D	8. C
9. B	9. D
10. D	10. C
11. B	11. D
12. C	12. A
13. D	13. A
14. A	14. B
15. C	15. E
16. A	16. D
17. B	17. D
18. B	18. D
19. A	19. E
20. B	20. E

Index

How to Receive Continuing Education Credits

The four individual modules of the *Lactation Specialist Self-Study Series* have been approved for continuing education hours/continuing education recognition points (CERPs)/contact hours from the following organizations:

Commission on Dietetic Registration (CDR): The credentialing agency for the American Dietetic Association.

Georgia Nurses Association (GNA): The Georgia Nurses Association is accredited as an Approver of Continuing Education in Nursing by the American Nurses Credentialing Center Commission on Accreditation.

International Board of Lactation Consultant Examiners (IBLCE): The International Board of Lactation Consultant Examiners is the credentialing agency for the International Lactation Consultant Association.

The individual purchasing the module(s) can apply for continuing education credits/contact hours/CERPs for any **one** or **all** of the four modules in the series. The following chart explains the credits approved by each organization for each of the four modules:

		CDR*	GNA	IBLCE
Module 1	*The Support of Breastfeeding*	15 CE Category II	18	18L Independent
Module 2	*The Process of Breastfeeding*	15 CE Category III	18	18L Independent
Module 3	*The Science of Breastfeeding*	23 CE Category III	27	27L Independent
Module 4	*The Management of Breastfeeding*	15 CE Category III	18	18L Independent

*The Commission on Dietetic Registration has approved all four modules for specialist CE approval for Board Certified Specialists in Pediatric Nutrition.

Procedure to Follow to Apply for Credits

Step 1   Remove the application for continuing education, answer sheet and evaluation from the back of the module. Do not lose the application form because it has been specially processed to identify originals packaged with each module and can only be replaced for a $25.00 fee accompanied by the original receipt of purchase. Photocopies of the application form will not be accepted. Only one application is needed to apply for credits from more than one organization. Complete the application for continuing education.

Step 2   Review the objectives for each section prior to reading the section or taking the pre-test. Take the pre-test and fill in your answers on the answer sheet for the section to be studied. You must complete the pre-test to obtain credits, although your score on the pre-test will not influence whether or not you obtain credits. Please answer the pre-test to the best of your ability because the score on the pre-test will be pooled with the scores of other applicants and used to assist the editors in identifying areas applicants are weak in and will be compared to your post-test to quantify the success of the module in enhancing learning.

After you have taken the pre-test and recorded your answers on the official answer sheet, read and study the section. Finally, complete the post-test and fill in the answers on the official answer sheet. **Only the answers on the post-test will be scored for continuing education**. You must receive a 70% correct on the post-test for each section in the module to obtain credit. If you score less than 70% on any one post-test of the module, you will be sent a listing of references pertinent to the section(s) you did not complete successfully and can re-apply for continuing education credits for a discounted fee of $1.00 per continuing education credit. Should this occur, you will be sent another answer sheet to use because photocopies of the answer sheets are not accepted.

Step 3   Complete the module evaluation after reading each section. The module evaluations will be analyzed and the information obtained used to improve and enhance the series. Send the module evaluation(s), official answer sheets(s) and check, money order or credit card information to ANC, Inc., 4833 McGahee Road, Evans, GA 30809.

Allow three weeks for processing. Rush processing is available for an extra $25.00: scoring and notification of credits to credentialing agencies will be completed within three business days of receiving your application and the rush processing fee.

Step 4   Upon successful completion of all the post-tests for a module, you will be sent a certificate of completion for each organization that you have requested credit from; your name will be forwarded to the appropriate credentialing organization, if appropriate; and a record will be maintained of your successful completion for five years. Requests for duplicate certificates can be honored for a processing fee of $10.00.

Module 2   The Process of Breastfeeding
APPLICATION FOR CONTINUING EDUCATION CREDITS

Name _____
as it will appear on certificate

Address _____
street, rural route, or post office box

City _____ State/Province _____ Zip code _____

Country_____

Daytime phone no. _____ e-mail _____
area code and number

Please complete the information for the organization(s) from which you are requesting credit:

Commission on Dietetic Registration   CE hours: ____ × $2.00 = _____

Are you a board certified specialist in pediatric nutrition?   Yes ____   No ____

Registration Number _____

Georgia Nurses Association   Contact hours: ____ × $2.00 = _____

SSN/SIN _____

International Board of Lactation   CERPs: ____ × $2.00 = _____
Consultant Examiners

SSN/SIN or IBLCE 9-digit ID number _____

Optional rush processing ($25.00 fee) _____

TOTAL _____

Checks, money orders, and credit cards accepted. No purchase orders.

____ MasterCard ____ Visa ____ American Express

Account Number _____ Expiration Date _____

Name as it appears on the card _____

Checks or money orders may be made out to **Augusta Nutrition Consultants, Inc. (ANC)** and sent with the evaluation and completed answer sheet to 4833 McGahee Road, Evans, GA 30809.

DO NOT SEND TO JONES AND BARTLETT PUBLISHERS.

Note: You must submit this **original** form to receive continuing education units. Photocopies cannot be accepted.

Evaluation
The Process of Breastfeeding

Please comment on the degree of content difficulty, effectiveness of learning method, and objectives for the following topics by putting a checkmark in the circle next to the response that best describes the material.

Preparing to Breastfeed

Content level	○ too high	○ appropriate	○ too low
Effectiveness of learning method	○ excellent/very good	○ good	○ fair/poor
Information	○ useful		○ not useful

Use the following key for the objectives and circle your response:

1 = STRONGLY MET   **2** = MET   **3** = SOMEWHAT MET   **4** = SOMEWHAT NOT MET   **5** = NOT MET

At the completion of this section, the learner will be able to do the following:

1. Identify three important questions to ask the mother in the prenatal period.   1 2 3 4 5

2. Assess the prenatal client's nipples and breasts for abnormalities that might interfere with function.   1 2 3 4 5

3. Identify types of nipple protractability, offering suggestions for prenatal and postpartum management of retracted or inverted nipples.   1 2 3 4 5

4. Instruct the prenatal and postpartum breastfeeding mother on proper nipple and breast care.   1 2 3 4 5

Feeding at the Breast

Content level	○ too high	○ appropriate	○ too low
Effectiveness of learning method	○ excellent/very good	○ good	○ fair/poor
Information	○ useful		○ not useful

Use the following key for the objectives and circle your response:

1 = STRONGLY MET   **2** = MET   **3** = SOMEWHAT MET   **4** = SOMEWHAT NOT MET   **5** = NOT MET

At the completion of this section, the learner will be able to do the following:

1. List three signs of an infant's readiness to breastfeed.   1 2 3 4 5

2. List three signs of a mother's readiness to breastfeed.   1 2 3 4 5

3. Describe two techniques for supporting the breast while breastfeeding.   1 2 3 4 5

4. Instruct the client on breastfeeding basics, including   1 2 3 4 5
   positioning, cueing, and latching techniques.

Breastfeeding Assessment

Content level	○ too high	○ appropriate	○ too low
Effectiveness of learning method	○ excellent/very good	○ good	○ fair/poor
Information	○ useful		○ not useful

Use the following key for the objectives and circle your response:

1 = STRONGLY MET   **2** = MET   **3** = SOMEWHAT MET   **4** = SOMEWHAT NOT MET   **5** = NOT MET

At the completion of this section, the learner will be able to do the following:

1. Assess the infant at breast for correct positioning, latch-on,   1 2 3 4 5
   sucking, and milk transfer.

2. State two anatomic characteristics specific to the infant that   1 2 3 4 5
   assist with breastfeeding.

3. Instruct the breastfeeding mother on how to assess audible   1 2 3 4 5
   swallowing while the infant is breastfeeding and explain the
   importance of this assessment.

4. Describe differences in expected stooling and urine patterns   1 2 3 4 5
   of the newborn and older infant.

5. List the steps to performing a digital suck assessment.   1 2 3 4 5

6. List three symptoms and signs in the infant that alert the   1 2 3 4 5
   clinician to intervene.

7. Describe two assessment tools that can be used to evaluate   1 2 3 4 5
   breastfeeding.

8. Describe two charting methods that can be useful in docu-   1 2 3 4 5
   menting encounters with breastfeeding women and their
   families.

Areolar and Nipple Tissue Structural Elements and Wound Healing

Content level	○ too high	○ appropriate	○ too low
Effectiveness of learning method	○ excellent/very good	○ good	○ fair/poor
Information	○ useful		○ not useful

Use the following key for the objectives and circle your response:

1 = STRONGLY MET   **2** = MET   **3** = SOMEWHAT MET   **4** = SOMEWHAT NOT MET   **5** = NOT MET

At the completion of this section, the learner will be able to do the following:

1. Identify the epidermis and dermis layers of skin and dis-   1 2 3 4 5
   cuss their functions.

2. Discuss the role of keratin in relation to the breast. 1 2 3 4 5

3. Discuss the roles of the sebaceous gland and sebum in relation to the breast and breastfeeding. 1 2 3 4 5

4. Discuss the role of tissue repair: dry wound healing versus moist wound healing. 1 2 3 4 5

5. Discuss the role nutrition plays in wound healing. 1 2 3 4 5

Nipple Soreness

Content level   ○ too high   ○ appropriate   ○ too low

Effectiveness of learning method   ○ excellent/very good   ○ good   ○ fair/poor

Information   ○ useful   ○ not useful

Use the following key for the objectives and circle your response:

1 = STRONGLY MET   **2** = MET   **3** = SOMEWHAT MET   **4** = SOMEWHAT NOT MET   **5** = NOT MET

At the completion of this section, the learner will be able to do the following:

1. Discuss prenatal preparation of the nipples. 1 2 3 4 5

2. Identify and discuss possible causes of sore nipples and offer suggestions for prevention and management. 1 2 3 4 5

3. Assess the infant at breast, recognize possible problem areas, and assist the mother to correct them without undermining her confidence in her ability to nourish her infant. 1 2 3 4 5

Breast-Related Problems

Content level   ○ too high   ○ appropriate   ○ too low

Effectiveness of learning method   ○ excellent/very good   ○ good   ○ fair/poor

Information   ○ useful   ○ not useful

Use the following key for the objectives and circle your response:

1 = STRONGLY MET   **2** = MET   **3** = SOMEWHAT MET   **4** = SOMEWHAT NOT MET   **5** = NOT MET

At the completion of this section, the learner will be able to do the following:

1. Recognize signs and symptoms of candidiasis and advise the breastfeeding mother of an appropriate plan of care. 1 2 3 4 5

2. Discuss the effects of herpes simplex virus on the breastfeeding relationship, offering recommendations for the lactating mother during a period of outbreak. 1 2 3 4 5

3. Identify various classifications of nipple function, offering ways to help manage ungraspable nipples for breastfeeding success. 1 2 3 4 5

4. Identify possible causes of nipple discharge and color variations in breastmilk. 1 2 3 4 5

5. Identify reasons for leakage of breastmilk, offering management recommendations.   1   2   3   4   5

6. Recognize the difference between two classifications of engorgement, offering recommendations for prevention and management.   1   2   3   4   5

7. Discuss possible causes of plugged ducts and provide recommendations for prevention and management.   1   2   3   4   5

8. Discuss possible causes of mastitis and provide recommendations for prevention and management.   1   2   3   4   5

9. Recognize signs and symptoms of an abscessed breast, offering recommendations for prevention and management.   1   2   3   4   5

10. Discuss the causes of a galactocele and management recommendations.   1   2   3   4   5

11. List signs of an overactive milk-ejection reflex and discuss management suggestions.   1   2   3   4   5

12. Discuss signs of an inhibited milk-ejection reflex, recognize possible causes, and offer management suggestions.   1   2   3   4   5

13. List factors contributing to an impaired milk supply and offer appropriate steps to assist the breastfeeding mother in increasing her milk supply.   1   2   3   4   5

Infant-Related Problems

Content level	○ too high	○ appropriate	○ too low
Effectiveness of learning method	○ excellent/very good	○ good	○ fair/poor
Information	○ useful		○ not useful

Use the following key for the objectives and circle your response:

1 = STRONGLY MET   **2** = MET   **3** = SOMEWHAT MET   **4** = SOMEWHAT NOT MET   **5** = NOT MET

At the completion of this section, the learner will be able to do the following:

1. Identify causes of breast refusal by the infant and provide recommendations for re-initiating and maintaining a successful breastfeeding relationship.   1   2   3   4   5

2. List possible causes of sucking difficulties and offer recommendations for management.   1   2   3   4   5

3. Discuss the possible side effects of the early introduction of artificial teats.   1   2   3   4   5

4. Discuss management suggestions for the infant presenting with nipple confusion.   1   2   3   4   5

5. Identify signs and symptoms of an infant displaying a weak suck and offer suggestions for management.   1   2   3   4   5

6. Recognize ankyloglossia and discuss possible treatment options, if indicated.   1 2 3 4 5

7. Discuss possible causes of tongue thrusting in the infant and offer recommendations for management.   1 2 3 4 5

8. Recognize signs of an infant presenting with a retracted or curled tongue and offer recommendations for management.   1 2 3 4 5

9. Discuss the characteristics displayed by an infant presenting with a tonic bite reflex and offer management suggestions.   1 2 3 4 5

10. Explain the effects of complementary and supplementary feeds in relation to milk production, milk intake, and sucking behavior of the breastfeeding infant.   1 2 3 4 5

Expression, Collection, and Storage of Breastmilk

Content level	○ too high	○ appropriate	○ too low
Effectiveness of learning method	○ excellent/very good	○ good	○ fair/poor
Information	○ useful		○ not useful

Use the following key for the objectives and circle your response:

1 = STRONGLY MET **2** = MET **3** = SOMEWHAT MET **4** = SOMEWHAT NOT MET **5** = NOT MET

At the completion of this section, the learner will be able to do the following:

1. Discuss and demonstrate the removal of breastmilk using the Marmet Technique for the manual expression of breastmilk.   1 2 3 4 5

2. Discuss the four basic categories of breast pumps available for the mechanical expression of breastmilk, stating when each may be appropriate.   1 2 3 4 5

3. Identify and discuss features and characteristics of the numerous breast pumps available on the market.   1 2 3 4 5

4. Provide instructions and recommendations for the mother using a breast pump.   1 2 3 4 5

5. Provide instructions and guidelines for the collection, storage, and preparation of expressed breastmilk.   1 2 3 4 5

6. Discuss the benefits of human milk banking.   1 2 3 4 5

Breastfeeding Accessories, Devices, and Supplemental Techniques

Content level	○ too high	○ appropriate	○ too low
Effectiveness of learning method	○ excellent/very good	○ good	○ fair/poor
Information	○ useful		○ not useful

Use the following key for the objectives and circle your response:

1 = STRONGLY MET   **2** = MET   **3** = SOMEWHAT MET   **4** = SOMEWHAT NOT MET   **5** = NOT MET

At the completion of this section, the learner will be able to do the following:

1. Identify situations in which the use of breast shells may benefit the breastfeeding mother and infant.   1 2 3 4 5

2. Discuss the dangers that accompany the use of nipple shields and provide instructions for correct usage if a nipple shield is used.   1 2 3 4 5

3. Identify a dimpled nipple and discuss the use of a dimple ring.   1 2 3 4 5

4. Provide recommendations to the mother who will be purchasing nursing bras and bra pads.   1 2 3 4 5

5. Provide data regarding creams and ointments for the breasts, discussing which type of creams and ointments to avoid and providing supporting rationale.   1 2 3 4 5

6. Discuss the role of the nursing supplemental device and idenrify situations in which the device could be beneficial.   1 2 3 4 5

7. Provide recommendations on the technique of finger feeding for nutritional supplementation.   1 2 3 4 5

8. Describe cup feeding as a technique for nutritional supplementation.   1 2 3 4 5

9. Describe the use of a periodontal syringe for providing nutritional supplementation.   1 2 3 4 5

10. Discuss the function of nursing stools and nursing pillows for the breastfeeding mother.   1 2 3 4 5

11. Discuss fashion options for the breastfeeding mother, offering recommendations.   1 2 3 4 5

Describe how the information presented is applicable to your practice:

Please tell us what you liked the best about the material:

Please tell us what you liked the least about the material:

Please evaluate the time required to complete the module when compared to the continuing education hours offered (check one):

     ○ more time required than hours awarded

     ○ approximately the same time required as hours awarded

     ○ less time required than hours awarded

Additional Comments:

Module 2 *The Process of Breastfeeding* Answer Sheet

Please use a number 2 pencil to mark your response.

Chapter 1 Section A Preparing to Breastfeed

	Pre-Test						Post-Test				
	a	b	c	d	e		a	b	c	d	e
1.	○	○	○	○	○	1.	○	○	○	○	○
2.	○	○	○	○	○	2.	○	○	○	○	○
3.	○	○	○	○	○	3.	○	○	○	○	○
4.	○	○	○	○	○	4.	○	○	○	○	○
5.	○	○	○	○	○	5.	○	○	○	○	○
6.	○	○	○	○	○	6.	○	○	○	○	○
7.	○	○	○	○	○	7.	○	○	○	○	○
8.	○	○	○	○	○	8.	○	○	○	○	○
9.	○	○	○	○	○	9.	○	○	○	○	○
10.	○	○	○	○	○	10.	○	○	○	○	○
11.	○	○	○	○	○	11.	○	○	○	○	○
12.	○	○	○	○	○	12.	○	○	○	○	○
13.	○	○	○	○	○	13.	○	○	○	○	○
14.	○	○	○	○	○	14.	○	○	○	○	○
15.	○	○	○	○	○	15.	○	○	○	○	○
16.	○	○	○	○	○	16.	○	○	○	○	○
17.	○	○	○	○	○	17.	○	○	○	○	○
18.	○	○	○	○	○	18.	○	○	○	○	○
19.	○	○	○	○	○	19.	○	○	○	○	○
20.	○	○	○	○	○	20.	○	○	○	○	○

Chapter 1 Section B Feeding at the Breast

	Pre-Test						Post-Test				
	a	b	c	d	e		a	b	c	d	e
1.	○	○	○	○	○	1.	○	○	○	○	○
2.	○	○	○	○	○	2.	○	○	○	○	○
3.	○	○	○	○	○	3.	○	○	○	○	○
4.	○	○	○	○	○	4.	○	○	○	○	○
5.	○	○	○	○	○	5.	○	○	○	○	○
6.	○	○	○	○	○	6.	○	○	○	○	○
7.	○	○	○	○	○	7.	○	○	○	○	○
8.	○	○	○	○	○	8.	○	○	○	○	○
9.	○	○	○	○	○	9.	○	○	○	○	○
10.	○	○	○	○	○	10.	○	○	○	○	○
11.	○	○	○	○	○	11.	○	○	○	○	○
12.	○	○	○	○	○	12.	○	○	○	○	○
13.	○	○	○	○	○	13.	○	○	○	○	○
14.	○	○	○	○	○	14.	○	○	○	○	○
15.	○	○	○	○	○	15.	○	○	○	○	○
16.	○	○	○	○	○	16.	○	○	○	○	○
17.	○	○	○	○	○	17.	○	○	○	○	○
18.	○	○	○	○	○	18.	○	○	○	○	○
19.	○	○	○	○	○	19.	○	○	○	○	○
20.	○	○	○	○	○	20.	○	○	○	○	○

Chapter 1 Section C Breastfeeding Assessment

	Pre-Test						**Post-Test**				
	a	b	c	d	e		a	b	c	d	e
1.	O	O	O	O	O	1.	O	O	O	O	O
2.	O	O	O	O	O	2.	O	O	O	O	O
3.	O	O	O	O	O	3.	O	O	O	O	O
4.	O	O	O	O	O	4.	O	O	O	O	O
5.	O	O	O	O	O	5.	O	O	O	O	O
6.	O	O	O	O	O	6.	O	O	O	O	O
7.	O	O	O	O	O	7.	O	O	O	O	O
8.	O	O	O	O	O	8.	O	O	O	O	O
9.	O	O	O	O	O	9.	O	O	O	O	O
10.	O	O	O	O	O	10.	O	O	O	O	O
11.	O	O	O	O	O	11.	O	O	O	O	O
12.	O	O	O	O	O	12.	O	O	O	O	O
13.	O	O	O	O	O	13.	O	O	O	O	O
14.	O	O	O	O	O	14.	O	O	O	O	O
15.	O	O	O	O	O	15.	O	O	O	O	O
16.	O	O	O	O	O	16.	O	O	O	O	O
17.	O	O	O	O	O	17.	O	O	O	O	O
18.	O	O	O	O	O	18.	O	O	O	O	O
19.	O	O	O	O	O	19.	O	O	O	O	O
20.	O	O	O	O	O	20.	O	O	O	O	O

Chapter 2 Section A Areolar and Nipple Tissue Structural Elements and Wound Healing

	Pre-Test						**Post-Test**				
	a	b	c	d	e		a	b	c	d	e
1.	O	O	O	O	O	1.	O	O	O	O	O
2.	O	O	O	O	O	2.	O	O	O	O	O
3.	O	O	O	O	O	3.	O	O	O	O	O
4.	O	O	O	O	O	4.	O	O	O	O	O
5.	O	O	O	O	O	5.	O	O	O	O	O
6.	O	O	O	O	O	6.	O	O	O	O	O
7.	O	O	O	O	O	7.	O	O	O	O	O
8.	O	O	O	O	O	8.	O	O	O	O	O
9.	O	O	O	O	O	9.	O	O	O	O	O
10.	O	O	O	O	O	10.	O	O	O	O	O
11.	O	O	O	O	O	11.	O	O	O	O	O
12.	O	O	O	O	O	12.	O	O	O	O	O
13.	O	O	O	O	O	13.	O	O	O	O	O
14.	O	O	O	O	O	14.	O	O	O	O	O
15.	O	O	O	O	O	15.	O	O	O	O	O
16.	O	O	O	O	O	16.	O	O	O	O	O
17.	O	O	O	O	O	17.	O	O	O	O	O
18.	O	O	O	O	O	18.	O	O	O	O	O
19.	O	O	O	O	O	19.	O	O	O	O	O
20.	O	O	O	O	O	20.	O	O	O	O	O

Chapter 2 Section B   Nipple Soreness

	Pre-Test						Post-Test				
	a	b	c	d	e		a	b	c	d	e
1.	O	O	O	O	O	1.	O	O	O	O	O
2.	O	O	O	O	O	2.	O	O	O	O	O
3.	O	O	O	O	O	3.	O	O	O	O	O
4.	O	O	O	O	O	4.	O	O	O	O	O
5.	O	O	O	O	O	5.	O	O	O	O	O
6.	O	O	O	O	O	6.	O	O	O	O	O
7.	O	O	O	O	O	7.	O	O	O	O	O
8.	O	O	O	O	O	8.	O	O	O	O	O
9.	O	O	O	O	O	9.	O	O	O	O	O
10.	O	O	O	O	O	10.	O	O	O	O	O
11.	O	O	O	O	O	11.	O	O	O	O	O
12.	O	O	O	O	O	12.	O	O	O	O	O
13.	O	O	O	O	O	13.	O	O	O	O	O
14.	O	O	O	O	O	14.	O	O	O	O	O
15.	O	O	O	O	O	15.	O	O	O	O	O
16.	O	O	O	O	O	16.	O	O	O	O	O
17.	O	O	O	O	O	17.	O	O	O	O	O
18.	O	O	O	O	O	18.	O	O	O	O	O
19.	O	O	O	O	O	19.	O	O	O	O	O
20.	O	O	O	O	O	20.	O	O	O	O	O

Chapter 2 Section C   Breast-Related Problems

	Pre-Test						Post-Test				
	a	b	c	d	e		a	b	c	d	e
1.	O	O	O	O	O	1.	O	O	O	O	O
2.	O	O	O	O	O	2.	O	O	O	O	O
3.	O	O	O	O	O	3.	O	O	O	O	O
4.	O	O	O	O	O	4.	O	O	O	O	O
5.	O	O	O	O	O	5.	O	O	O	O	O
6.	O	O	O	O	O	6.	O	O	O	O	O
7.	O	O	O	O	O	7.	O	O	O	O	O
8.	O	O	O	O	O	8.	O	O	O	O	O
9.	O	O	O	O	O	9.	O	O	O	O	O
10.	O	O	O	O	O	10.	O	O	O	O	O
11.	O	O	O	O	O	11.	O	O	O	O	O
12.	O	O	O	O	O	12.	O	O	O	O	O
13.	O	O	O	O	O	13.	O	O	O	O	O
14.	O	O	O	O	O	14.	O	O	O	O	O
15.	O	O	O	O	O	15.	O	O	O	O	O
16.	O	O	O	O	O	16.	O	O	O	O	O
17.	O	O	O	O	O	17.	O	O	O	O	O
18.	O	O	O	O	O	18.	O	O	O	O	O
19.	O	O	O	O	O	19.	O	O	O	O	O
20.	O	O	O	O	O	20.	O	O	O	O	O

Chapter 2 Section D   Infant-Related Problems

	Pre-Test					Post-Test				
	a	b	c	d	e	a	b	c	d	e
1.	○	○	○	○	○	○	○	○	○	○
2.	○	○	○	○	○	○	○	○	○	○
3.	○	○	○	○	○	○	○	○	○	○
4.	○	○	○	○	○	○	○	○	○	○
5.	○	○	○	○	○	○	○	○	○	○
6.	○	○	○	○	○	○	○	○	○	○
7.	○	○	○	○	○	○	○	○	○	○
8.	○	○	○	○	○	○	○	○	○	○
9.	○	○	○	○	○	○	○	○	○	○
10.	○	○	○	○	○	○	○	○	○	○
11.	○	○	○	○	○	○	○	○	○	○
12.	○	○	○	○	○	○	○	○	○	○
13.	○	○	○	○	○	○	○	○	○	○
14.	○	○	○	○	○	○	○	○	○	○
15.	○	○	○	○	○	○	○	○	○	○
16.	○	○	○	○	○	○	○	○	○	○
17.	○	○	○	○	○	○	○	○	○	○
18.	○	○	○	○	○	○	○	○	○	○
19.	○	○	○	○	○	○	○	○	○	○
20.	○	○	○	○	○	○	○	○	○	○

Chapter 3 Section A   Expression, Collection, and Storage of Breastmilk

	Pre-Test					Post-Test				
	a	b	c	d	e	a	b	c	d	e
1.	○	○	○	○	○	○	○	○	○	○
2.	○	○	○	○	○	○	○	○	○	○
3.	○	○	○	○	○	○	○	○	○	○
4.	○	○	○	○	○	○	○	○	○	○
5.	○	○	○	○	○	○	○	○	○	○
6.	○	○	○	○	○	○	○	○	○	○
7.	○	○	○	○	○	○	○	○	○	○
8.	○	○	○	○	○	○	○	○	○	○
9.	○	○	○	○	○	○	○	○	○	○
10.	○	○	○	○	○	○	○	○	○	○
11.	○	○	○	○	○	○	○	○	○	○
12.	○	○	○	○	○	○	○	○	○	○
13.	○	○	○	○	○	○	○	○	○	○
14.	○	○	○	○	○	○	○	○	○	○
15.	○	○	○	○	○	○	○	○	○	○
16.	○	○	○	○	○	○	○	○	○	○
17.	○	○	○	○	○	○	○	○	○	○
18.	○	○	○	○	○	○	○	○	○	○
19.	○	○	○	○	○	○	○	○	○	○
20.	○	○	○	○	○	○	○	○	○	○

Chapter 3 Section B   Breastfeeding Accessories,
Devices, and Supplemental Techniques

	Pre-Test						**Post-Test**				
	a	b	c	d	e		a	b	c	d	e
1.	O	O	O	O	O	1.	O	O	O	O	O
2.	O	O	O	O	O	2.	O	O	O	O	O
3.	O	O	O	O	O	3.	O	O	O	O	O
4.	O	O	O	O	O	4.	O	O	O	O	O
5.	O	O	O	O	O	5.	O	O	O	O	O
6.	O	O	O	O	O	6.	O	O	O	O	O
7.	O	O	O	O	O	7.	O	O	O	O	O
8.	O	O	O	O	O	8.	O	O	O	O	O
9.	O	O	O	O	O	9.	O	O	O	O	O
10.	O	O	O	O	O	10.	O	O	O	O	O
11.	O	O	O	O	O	11.	O	O	O	O	O
12.	O	O	O	O	O	12.	O	O	O	O	O
13.	O	O	O	O	O	13.	O	O	O	O	O
14.	O	O	O	O	O	14.	O	O	O	O	O
15.	O	O	O	O	O	15.	O	O	O	O	O
16.	O	O	O	O	O	16.	O	O	O	O	O
17.	O	O	O	O	O	17.	O	O	O	O	O
18.	O	O	O	O	O	18.	O	O	O	O	O
19.	O	O	O	O	O	19.	O	O	O	O	O
20.	O	O	O	O	O	20.	O	O	O	O	O